Clinical Nursing Skills
at a Glance

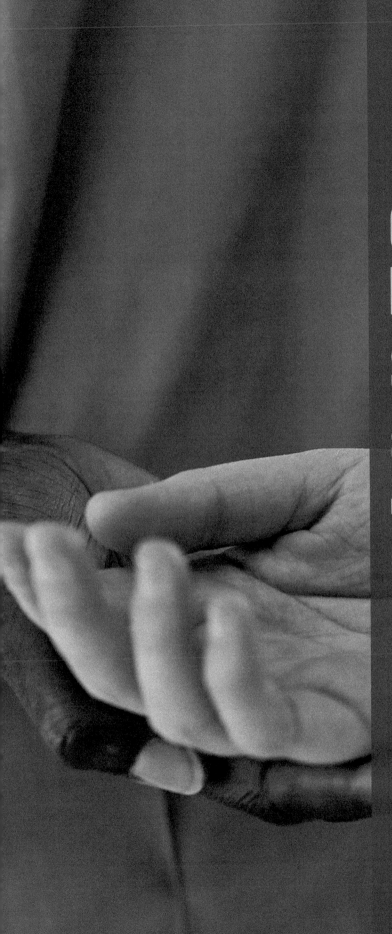

Clinical
Nursing
Skills
at a Glance

Edited by

Sarah Curr
King's College London
London

Carol Fordham-Clarke
King's College London
London

Series Editor: Ian Peate

WILEY Blackwell

This edition first published 2022
© 2022 John Wiley & Sons Ltd

The right of Carol Fordham-Clarke and Sarah Curr to be identified as the authors of the editorial material in this work has been asserted in accordance with law.

Registered Offices
John Wiley & Sons, Inc., 111 River Street, Hoboken, NJ 07030, USA

John Wiley & Sons Ltd, The Atrium, Southern Gate, Chichester, West Sussex, PO19 8SQ, UK

Editorial Office
9600 Garsington Road, Oxford, OX4 2DQ, UK

For details of our global editorial offices, customer services, and more information about Wiley products visit us at www.wiley.com.

Wiley also publishes its books in a variety of electronic formats and by print-on-demand. Some content that appears in standard print versions of this book may not be available in other formats.

Library of Congress Cataloging-in-Publication data applied for

PB ISBN: 9781119035909

Cover Design: Wiley
Cover Image: © PeopleImages/Getty Images

Set in 9.5/11.5pt Minion by Straive, Pondicherry, India
Printed and bound by CPI Group (UK) Ltd, Croydon, CR0 4YY

C9781119035909_080222

Contents

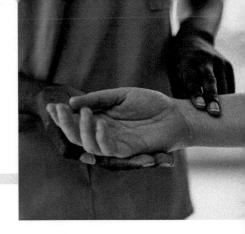

Part 11 Endocrine skills 157

Part 12 Circulatory Skills 161

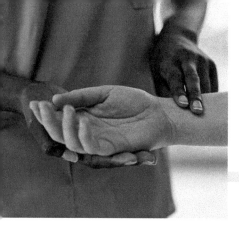

List of contributors

Tiago Horta Reis da Silva MSc, MBA, MScTCM, PGDipSFC, PGDipHE, PGCertHE, BSc (HONS) (Nurs), BSc (HONS) (TCM), RN, FHEA, MBAcC
Lecturer in Nursing Education, Florence Nightingale Faculty of Nursing, Midwifery and Palliative Care, King's College London
London, United Kingdom

Rhiannon Eley RN, MSc, DTN, PGCert Clin.Ed, FHEA
Sister, Urgent Care Centre, Princess Grace Hospital, London, UK
PhD Candidate, King's College London, London, UK

Joanna De Souza RN, MSc, PATHE, RNT, AKC
Senior Lecturer, Florence Nightingale Faculty of Nursing, Midwifery and Palliative Care.
King's College London
London, UK

Dr Alison Gallagher FHEA
Senior Lecturer, Programme Director MSc Advanced Clinical Practice
School of Nursing, Midwifery and Social Work,
Canterbury Christ Church University
Chatham, UK

Kate Brown MSc, PGDipHE, BA(hons), RGN
Faculty Director for Simulation and Clinical Skills
Canterbury Christ Church University
Canterbury, United Kingdom

Karen Fawkes MSc, BSc, PGCE, FHEA, RGN
Teaching Fellow, Florence Nightingale Faculty of Nursing, Midwifery and Palliative Care, King's College London
London, United Kingdom

Lucy Tyler, RN, BSc, MSc, FHEA
Senior Lecturer in Adult Nursing
School of life and health sciences
University of Roehampton
London, United Kingdom

Helen B McInnes RN MSc
Nurse Specialist – Cancer Information, Dimbleby Cancer Care, Guy's Cancer Centre
Guy's and St Thomas' NHS Foundation Trust
London, UK

Acknowledgement

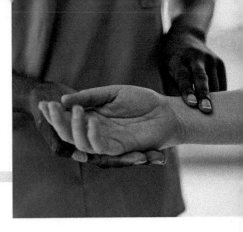

This book owes a great deal of thanks to many people. Firstly, to our colleagues at the Chantler SaIL centre who always helped to ensure we could have time, space, and equipment to secure our images, despite a global pandemic. Specific thanks goes to

- Amy Dines
- David Easton
- James Gaydon
- Courtney Woolgar

Secondly to Karen Fawkes and Tiago Horta Reis Da Silva who gave their time whenever asked. We are greatly appreciative.

To the team at Wiley, specifically Louise Barneston and Ashley Alliano, who supported us to get to publication.

Finally, to our friends and family, thank you for your endurance.

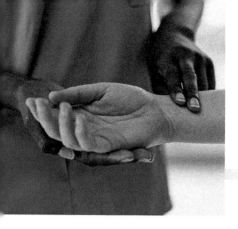

About the companion website

This book is accompanied by a companion website.

www.wiley.com/go/clinicalnursingskills

This website includes:

- Scenarios
- MCQs

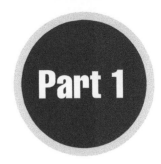

Part 1

Chapter

1 Introduction: the setup of this book and how to use it

This book is separated into 12 key sections with each section related to a system of the body. The exceptions to this are Chapter 2 (Principles of Skills) and Chapter 3 (Mandatory Skills). The principles of skills highlight key considerations for your healthcare practice, with the mandatory skills focusing on key skills required prior to entering the clinical environment to ensure safe practice. As such, these sections are intended to be read first.

Within this book each page is presented in an easy-to-follow double-page spread. This double page provides written content and tables, figures, and photos, which add a visual context and support.

The United Kingdom (UK) National Health Service Knowledge and Skills Framework (KSF) (NHS Employers 2019) was key in the development of this book due to its focus on the necessary knowledge and skills required to enable quality care provision. As such, each chapter provides both knowledge and skill, thereby ensuring an evidence-based approach to each skill. Each chapter has a brief background section where knowledge is provided with guidance for the procedure. The skill is then outlined in the sections on influencing factors, equipment and procedure. Each chapter also has a red flags section for specific signs and concerns to look for as well as actions to take.

The skills in this book have the potential to be used for all healthcare professionals but there is a recognition that much of these skills will be undertaken by the nursing workforce. As such this book provides skills that align with the UK Nursing & Midwifery's Council (NMC) *Standards of Proficiency for Registered Nurses* (2018). Throughout the book, and weaved across each chapter, are the core platforms:

- Being an accountable professional.
- Promoting health and ill health.
- Assessing need and planning care.
- Providing and evaluating care.
- Leading and managing care and working in teams.
- Improving safety and quality of care.
- Coordinating care.

We feel that whist skills have changed to incorporate the complex care delivery now required, these skills reflect commonly performed procedures in practice as well as those highlighted within the annex of the above publication (NMC 2018). We would also like to emphasise that all these skills require training and an assessment of competence and that this book is intended as a learning adjunct to clinical practice. Prior to performing each skill, you must have been assessed and deemed competent, thus having the necessary knowledge and skills to undertake the procedure.

Do use this book to inform your clinical practice, always ensuring that you use it whist following local and national policies and guidance. The purpose of this book is to provide a quick visual approach to essential healthcare skills and as such should be supplemented by material providing detailed theory underpinning the skills. However the knowledge gained within these chapters can be further consolidated within our online complementary package, which is available in www.wiley.com/go/clinicalnursingskills. This will test your knowledge through quizzes and case studies to ensure further preparedness for practice. Enjoy!

References

NHS Employers (2019) *Simplified Knowledge and Skills Framework.* https://www.nhsemployers.org/SimplifiedKSF (accessed 5 December 2020).

Nursing & Midwifery Council (2018). *Standards of Proficiency for Registered Nurses.* London: Nursing & Midwifery Council.

Principles of skills

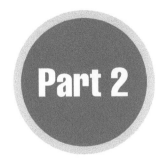

Part 2

Chapters

2 Care planning and the nursing process

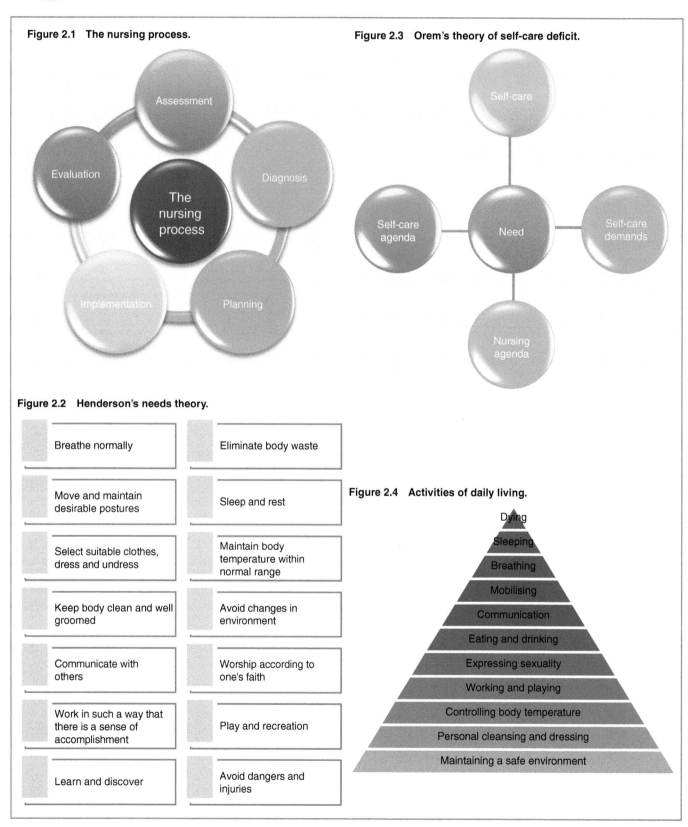

Figure 2.1   The nursing process.

- Assessment
- Diagnosis
- Planning
- Implementation
- Evaluation

The nursing process

Figure 2.3   Orem's theory of self-care deficit.

- Self-care
- Self-care agenda
- Need
- Self-care demands
- Nursing agenda

Figure 2.2   Henderson's needs theory.

Breathe normally	Eliminate body waste
Move and maintain desirable postures	Sleep and rest
Select suitable clothes, dress and undress	Maintain body temperature within normal range
Keep body clean and well groomed	Avoid changes in environment
Communicate with others	Worship according to one's faith
Work in such a way that there is a sense of accomplishment	Play and recreation
Learn and discover	Avoid dangers and injuries

Figure 2.4   Activities of daily living.

- Dying
- Sleeping
- Breathing
- Mobilising
- Communication
- Eating and drinking
- Expressing sexuality
- Working and playing
- Controlling body temperature
- Personal cleansing and dressing
- Maintaining a safe environment

Clinical Nursing Skills at a Glance, First Edition. Edited by Sarah Curr and Carol Fordham-Clarke.
© 2022 John Wiley & Sons Ltd. Published 2022 by John Wiley & Sons Ltd.
Companion website: www.wiley.com/go/clinicalnursingskills

Background

Care planning has been a core component of health and social care for many years and was first introduced as part of the nursing process by Ida Jean Orlando (1961). This four-stage process focused on the initial assessment, care planning, implementation, and then evaluation of the care delivery (Orlando 1961). This is intended as an ongoing, circular, activity (Figure 2.1) until care is no longer required and the patient is discharged from the service.

Since its introduction, the nursing process has evolved, with diagnosis being added by Gebbie and Lavin in 1973. The term diagnosis in nursing has long been debated due to its medical undertones, with Levine coining the term "trophicognosis" (Levine 1965) to replace diagnosis. This is because the term means the art and knowledge of nursing (Levine 1965) and refers to the use of information from the assessment and our pre-existing knowledge, which allows us to judge the need and thus create an individualised care plan.

Whichever the term used, the provision of individualised care is key to ensuring that high-quality care that places the patient at the centre is delivered. This also involves recognising that care planning, where possible, should involve the patient and the healthcare professional working together to plan care and set goals that are both desirable and achievable (NHSE 2016).

Influencing Factors

- When patients cannot be involved in the care planning, such as in an emergency or with unconscious patients, ensure that you act in their best interests. This will involve establishing if there is an advanced care plan or "living will". You will also need to establish if legal power of attorney has been granted to an individual and to ensure that person is involved in the process.
- Care planning may well differ across settings, but regardless of the setting there will be an opportunity to document the care plan, either digitally or written. This must be done to ensure continuity of care and a timely evaluation.

Professional Approach

- When assessing patients, ensure that they are fully informed by explaining the rationale of the assessment and how it will ensure care delivery that meets their individual needs.
- While you may be undertaking an individual assessment, planning care will most likely involve other members of the multidisciplinary team (MDT). Ensure that all members of the MDT are involved that are required, undertaking referrals where necessary.

Equipment

- Appropriate assessment paperwork.
- Patient's notes.
- Care planning paperwork.

Procedure – Assessment

This will involve using the relevant assessment documents within your clinical area. The questions asked may reflect Henderson's needs theory (Henderson 1966) (Figure 2.2), Orem's theory of self-care deficit (Orem 2001) (Figure 2.3), or Roper, Logan & Tierney's Activities of Daily Living model (Roper et al. 1980) (Figure 2.4). All these models focus on the fact that nursing care is provided while the patient cannot self-care or meet their daily needs.

Procedure – Diagnosis

- The diagnosis involves considering what has been observed and what information has been given during the initial assessment to identify the problem.
- The diagnosis focuses on key characteristics that enable the nursing diagnosis to be made.
- It is the diagnosis, or diagnoses, that inform the care plan.

Procedure – Care Planning

- More than one care plan may well need to be created to ensure that the patient's individualised needs are met.
- Care plan charts will most likely be available in your clinical area but the key elements to consider are:
  - What is the issue to be addressed?
  - What interventions will resolve this issue?
  - When would be it be appropriate to evaluate care?

Procedure – Implementation

- This is your ongoing care for the patient.
- Essentially by performing a thorough assessment, diagnosis and care plan, appropriate, necessary, person-centred care should be delivered.

Procedure – Evaluation

- This is when you review the care plan and determine if the initial issue has now resolved, remained the same, or worsened.
- Essentially the evaluation will then lead to an assessment and continuation of the process.

Red Flag

- ➤ If the patient becomes unresponsive during initial assessment the BLS (Basic Life Support) algorithm and the A–E (airway, breathing, circulation, disability, exposure) assessment should be used.
- ➤ A holistic assessment may take time as well as several discussions, depending on the patient's condition and priorities of care.

References

Gebbie, K. and Lavin, M.A. (1973). Classifying nursing diagnoses. *The American Journal of Nursing* 74 (2): 250–253.

Henderson, V. (1966). *The Nature of Nursing*. New York: Macmillian.

Levine, M.E. (1965). Trophicognosis: an alternative to nursing diagnosis. *ANA Clinical Conferences* 2: 55–70.

NHS England (2016). *Personalised Care and Support Planning Handbook: The Journey to Person Centred Care*. NHS England: Leeds.

Orem, D. (2001). *Nursing: Concepts of Practice*. St Louis: Mosby.

Orlando, I.J. (1961). *The Dynamic Nurse-Patient Relationship, Function, Process and Principles*. New York: Putnam Press.

Roper, N., Logan, W., and Tierney, A.J. (1980). *The Elements of Nursing*. London: Churchill Livingstone.

3 Communication – fundamentals

Table 3.1 Examples of paraphrasing.

	Patient	Healthcare worker
Summarising	"I'm the bread winner, I'm not sure what will happen to my family."	"You are worried about how your family with cope financially."
Interpreting	"I'm waiting on the results. I've been waiting a while."	"You're worried about when you're getting your results."

Table 3.2 Clarification questions.

"So, what you're saying is. . .?"

"Am I correct in understanding that. . .?"

"So what you mean by that is. . .?"

"What I'm hearing is. . ., is that correct?"

"I'm not quite sure I follow, could you give me more details?"

Table 3.3 SOLER – a tool to build rapport Identified by Egan (2014).

S	**Sit** at a comfortable angle and distance
O	Maintain an **open** posture, i.e. uncrossing legs and arms
L	**Lean** forward appropriately to show engagement
E	Maintain **eye** contact. The healthcare professional must be aware of when this might not be culturally appropriate
R	Maintain a relaxed posture. This will help with building rapport and trust.

Clinical Nursing Skills at a Glance, First Edition. Edited by Sarah Curr and Carol Fordham-Clarke.
© 2022 John Wiley & Sons Ltd. Published 2022 by John Wiley & Sons Ltd.
Companion website: www.wiley.com/go/clinicalnursingskills

Background

Communication is undertaken with every social interaction and effective communication is affected by how the message is sent and how it is received (Gates et al. 2003). Communication is recognised by the Nursing & Midwifery Council as an essential skill (2018) and involves written, verbal, and non-verbal communication, with patients/clients/service users, relatives, carers, and other members of the immediate and wider multi-professional team.

Influencing Factors

How we communicate depends on the client group we are communicating with and can change when:

- Communicating with people from different cultures.
- Communicating with people who speak different languages.
- Communicating with those with learning disabilities.
- Communicating with children.
- Communicating with those with dementia and/or delirium and other neurological impairments.
- There is a lack of time – it will be apparent by your body language if you feel that you do not have time for the interaction. This can be mitigated by providing a more suitable time for the conversation.

Professional Approach

In nursing how we communicate will impact upon the therapeutic relationship and trust built between the professional and the patient. How we communicate should be considered at the beginning of each episode of care and must be open, honest and non-judgemental. There are numerous factors that we must consider:

- The environment – where is the best place for this conversation?
- Physical discomfort, e.g. pain – consider giving analgesia before the conversation.
- Psychological discomfort, e.g. anxiety – adjusting body language, volume, articulation, pitch, emphasis and rate (VAPER) (Nelson-Jones 2014) of verbal communication can help here.
- Emotional discomfort, e.g. grief.
- Physical impairments, e.g. sight or hearing impairment– consider proximity, visual aids.
- Jargon – avoid professional language the patient may be unfamiliar with as this will create an additional barrier.

Procedure: Verbal Communication

Verbal communication can be face-to-face, over the telephone, or through other media forms, e.g. Facetime, Skype:

- Listening – this is a key aspect of verbal communication as it shows we are attentive and interested in the message being conveyed. It also demonstrates that we receive the message, understand it, support the person we are communicating with, and thus validate the message being delivered.
- Active listening involves paraphrasing, where the key points are repeated back to show that the correct message is being received (Table 3.1).
- Active listening can also involve the use of paralanguage such as: "mmh", "yes", "uh-huh", to show that you are listening.
- Verbal communication may initially start with closed questions, such as "Were you inside or outside?", which can be used at the outset, and open questions, such as "How did you feel when that happened?", to build rapport and engagement.

- Open questions are then used to gain more detailed information and insight into how the person is feeling.
- When communicating verbally there are other factors to consider. VAPER can help us to reflect on our communication in the moment and adjust accordingly (Nelson-Jones 2014).
- If you are not fully following the message it is acceptable to ask for clarification. Table 3.2 provides examples of clarification questions.

Procedure: Non-verbal Communication

- Non-verbal communication involves body language, our gestures, and dress (e.g. uniform), and can also be impacted by our height, gender, and scent, which some may find intimidating.
- As healthcare professionals work in closer proximity than is socially comfortable we need to be aware of our non-verbal communication and utilise this method of communication to demonstrate our care and compassion.
- Egan's acronym SOLER (Egan 2014) can be a useful tool to use initially to build rapport (Table 3.3).
- Communication is often split into three Cs, represented as 55/38/7 (Mehrabian 1972): 55% of communication occurs through body language, 33% through tone of voice, and 7% through the actual words said. Although this is often contested, it is certainly worth considering when engaged in communication.
- In some instances, therapeutic use of silence is also required, allowing the person time to express their message.

Written Communication

- Written communication can be used where there is an impairment impacting on the verbal message being received.
- It can also be used when professionals need to communicate with each other, i.e. via emails or in multidisciplinary notes.
- Written communication needs to be clear, concise, and legible. The key points need to be emphasised, jargon must be avoided, and the patient needs to be comfortable with, and able to use, this method.

Red Flags

- ☛ New dysphasia or dysarthria.
- ☛ New or sudden onset of confusion.
- ☛ Decrease in level of consciousness.
- ☛ Changes in behaviour following injury.

References

Egan, G. (2014). *The Skilled Helper: A Problem Management and Opportunity Development Approach to Helping*, 10e. California: Brooks-Cole.

Gates, B., Ellis, R.B., and Kenworthy, N. (2003). *Interpersonal Communication in Nursing: Theory and Practice*, 2e. Churchill Livingstone.

Mehrabian, A. (1972). *Nonverbal Communication*. Chicago: Aldine-Atherton.

Nelson-Jones, R. (2014). *Nelson-Jones' Theory and Practice of Counselling and Psychotherapy*, 6e. London: Sage Publications.

Nursing & Midwifery Council (2018). *Standards for Competence for Registered Nurses*. London: Nursing & Midwifery Council.

4 Record keeping

Figure 4.1 Mixing opinion and fact.

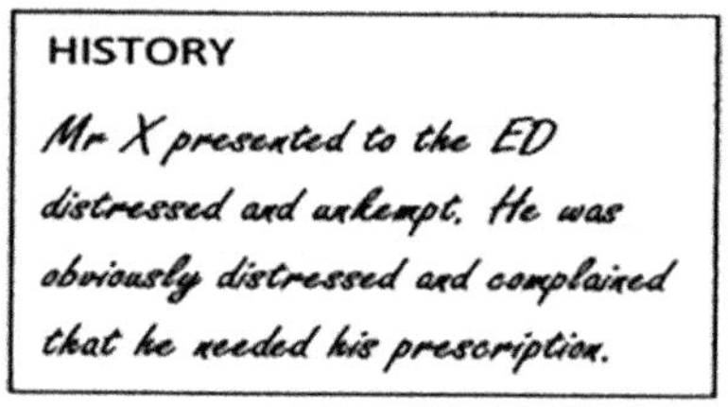

> HISTORY
>
> Mr X presented to the ED distressed and unkempt. He was obviously distressed and complained that he needed his prescription.

Figure 4.2 Illegible writing.

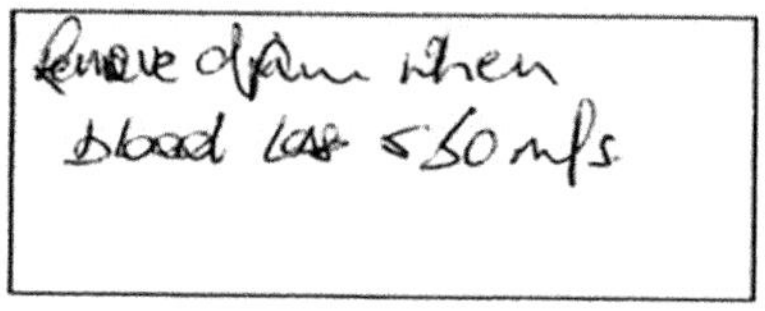

> Remove drain when blood loss ≤ 50 mls

Figure 4.3 Removing an error.

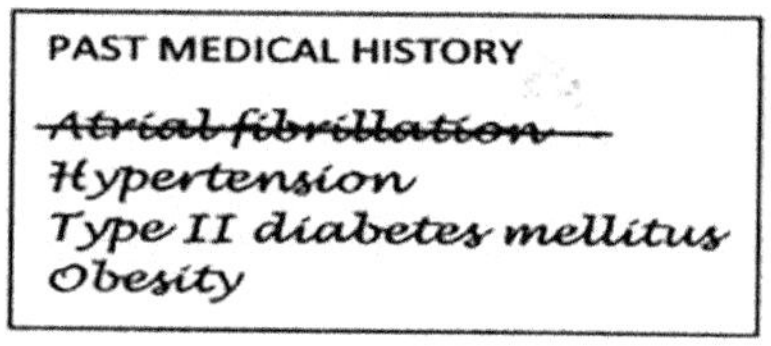

> PAST MEDICAL HISTORY
>
> ~~Atrial fibrillation~~
> Hypertension
> Type II diabetes mellitus
> Obesity

Figure 4.4 Designation and signature.

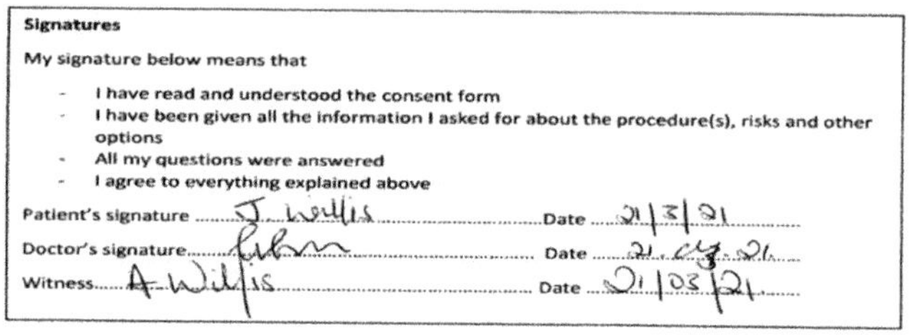

> Signatures
>
> My signature below means that
> - I have read and understood the consent form
> - I have been given all the information I asked for about the procedure(s), risks and other options
> - All my questions were answered
> - I agree to everything explained above
>
> Patient's signature ...... J. Wallis ...... Date 21/3/21
> Doctor's signature .... Date 21.03.21
> Witness ...... A. Willis ...... Date 21/03/21

Figure 4.5 Counter-signature.

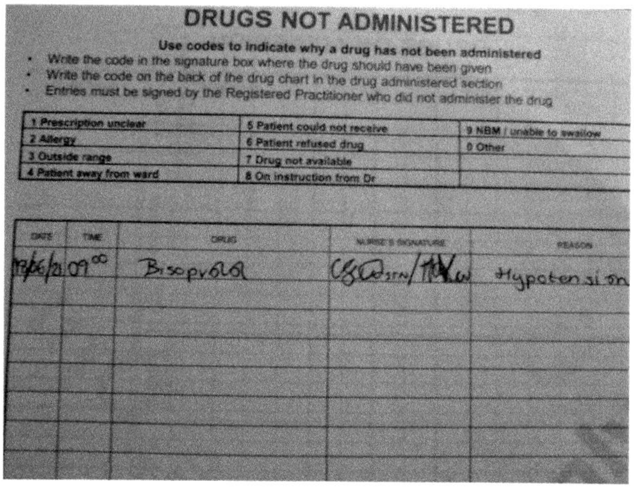

> DRUGS NOT ADMINISTERED
>
> Use codes to indicate why a drug has not been administered
> - Write the code in the signature box where the drug should have been given
> - Write the code on the back of the drug chart in the drug administered section
> - Entries must be signed by the Registered Practitioner who did not administer the drug

1 Prescription unclear	5 Patient could not receive	9 NBM / unable to swallow
2 Allergy	6 Patient refused drug	0 Other
3 Outside range	7 Drug not available	
4 Patient away from ward	8 On instruction from Dr	

DATE	TIME	DRUG	NURSE'S SIGNATURE	REASON
19/06/21	09:00	Bisoprolol	CG srn / ABW	Hypotension

Clinical Nursing Skills at a Glance, First Edition. Edited by Sarah Curr and Carol Fordham-Clarke.
© 2022 John Wiley & Sons Ltd. Published 2022 by John Wiley & Sons Ltd.
Companion website: www.wiley.com/go/clinicalnursingskills

Background

- Part 10 of the Nursing & Midwifery Council Code (NMC 2018) requires clear and accurate records to be kept.
- Record keeping is a key part of our communication within the interdisciplinary and multidisciplinary team (RCN 2017).
- Record keeping allows for communication of assessment, care planning, interventions, treatments, and evaluation.
- Poor record keeping has been linked to poor care and raised patient safety concerns (Francis 2013).
- While record keeping is key to providing continuity of care it should also be noted that any document can become a legal document once requested by the court (Dimond 2015).

Influencing Factors

- Critically unwell and/or hypovolaemic patients.
- Those who are agitated, confused or confrontational.
- Those in status epilepticus or having regular seizures.
- Needle phobia.

Professional Approach

- Time pressures – these pressures can result in documentation being delayed and thus it will not be as accurate as when recorded directly after the fact.
- Time pressures – these pressures can also cause handwriting to be illegible and result in typographic errors when using electronic records.
- Insufficient training on the documentation used can result in mistakes and/or omissions.
- Healthcare workers must remain up to date with training on record keeping, data collection, and storage and be aware of legal requirements about these.

Equipment

- The correct document to record the specific actions taken.
- Access codes may also be required.

Procedure – Standard Documentation

- Ensure that documentation is performed as soon after the fact as possible (RCN 2017).
- Avoid unnecessary abbreviations or abbreviations that could have multiple meanings, e.g. MS could refer to multiple sclerosis or mitral stenosis.
- Avoid unnecessary and/or inappropriate comments, such as mixing opinion and fact (Dimond 2015) (Figure 4.1).
- Avoid slang, jargon, derogatory, and any other comments that could be classed as unprofessional.
- Provide accurate and concise details of the intervention.
- Provide details on any future care required, i.e. next dressing change, evaluation of current care.
- Read through the work and ascertain if it would be understandable to the person who was provided with care (RCN 2017).
- Ensure that it is legible (Figure 4.2).
- If any errors are noted on written documentation, cross through the words with a single line (Figure 4.3).
- Provide date, time, and location of intervention.
- Provide designation and signature (Figure 4.4).
- Ensure a counter-signature is provided where required (Figure 4.5).

Procedure – Writing a Statement

You can be asked to write a statement as a witness to an incident, if you are under investigation, if you are raising a concern, or if you have a grievance. Professional bodies provide guidance and support on how to write individual statements but below are some key points:

- Provide your name, position, date, and subject heading – this includes any reference numbers.
- Highlight what this is connected to and the date and time of the incident. The introduction should also state your role in the incident.
- Provide a clear and full description of what occurred and when. Providing a clear account of an event can be challenging if a significant amount of time has elapsed. It is recommended that if you are involved in an incident that concerns you, you raise the concern and write the statement at that time.
- Highlight who was involved – this may include other colleagues, patients, family members, friends, significant others, and other members of the general public.
- Highlight any other factors that could have impacted on care provision such as short staffing, acuity of patients, caseload, any additional responsibilities.
- If possible, leave for one to two days before re-reading and submitting to the relevant personnel.
- If keeping an electronic copy, make sure it is encrypted.

Red Flag

- Patient safety should always be ensured before documentation.
- If you cannot read the patient's records, this needs to be escalated and the person involved will need to rewrite to ensure safe, effective, care provision.
- If care is not recorded, either written, typed, or in a voice file, it will be considered as not undertaken. This can result in duplication, which can be detrimental to patient care, e.g. medication administration.

References

Dimond, B. (2015). *Legal Aspects of Nursing*, 7e. Harlow: Pearson.

Francis, R. (2013). *The Mid Staffordshire NHS Foundation Trust Public Inquiry*. London: The Stationary Office.

Nursing & Midwifery Council (2018). *Professional Standards and Practice of Behaviour for Nurse, Midwives and Nursing Associates*. London: Nursing & Midwifery Council.

Royal College of Nursing (2017). *Record Keeping the Facts*. London: Royal College of Nursing.

5 Communication – de-escalation

Table 5.1 Signs of aggression.

Early signs of aggression	Danger signs of aggression
Prolonged eye contact	Continual staring; this will be at the intended target
Darkening of facial colour	Facial colour pales
Invasion of person space	Stance changes from square to side-on
Speaking loudly or yelling	Disengages from the conversation, may not be speaking
Intrusive or threatening gestures	Fist clenching and unclenching

Figure 5.1 Invasion of personal space.

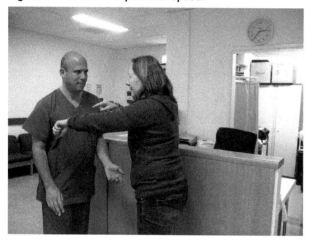

Figure 5.2 Calm, confident, and non-threatening approach.

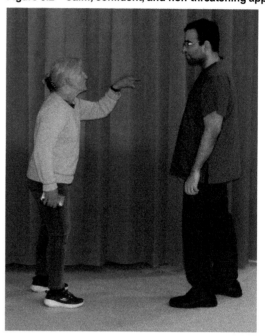

Figure 5.3 Showing concern and support.

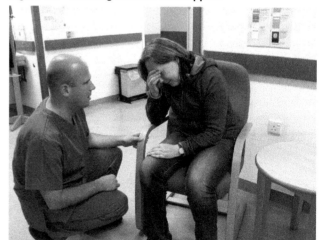

Clinical Nursing Skills at a Glance, First Edition. Edited by Sarah Curr and Carol Fordham-Clarke.
© 2022 John Wiley & Sons Ltd. Published 2022 by John Wiley & Sons Ltd.
Companion website: www.wiley.com/go/clinicalnursingskills

Background

In healthcare, patients, relatives, and significant others often experience heightened emotions, due to pain, anxiety, grief, physical impairments, and confusion. These heightened emotions can present in different ways and can potentially produce aggressive behaviour. Healthcare professionals are required to care for their patients, and this includes supporting them during these times of heightened emotion (Nursing & Midwifery Council 2018). To provide support during these instances, healthcare workers need to be trained in de-escalation skills and techniques (NICE 2015). NICE (2015) recognises that this training should include:

- Recognition of the early signs of anger (Table 5.1).
- Providing an understanding into the causes of aggression.
- Use of verbal and non-verbal techniques to distract and relax the patient.
- Responding to anger appropriately and in accordance with professional and legal frameworks.

It is important to remember that there are some instances where certain behaviours could be mistaken for signs of aggression. These could be:

- People who are shouting – this could be due to a loud environment or even a hearing impairment which could be chronic or from a new injury.
- People invading personal space – this could be due to the above reasons and they could also be seeking reassurance (Figure 5.1).
- Hypoglycaemia, which can cause people to display signs of aggression. Checking records and taking a full history can help avoid such errors.

Influencing Factors

- People who are under stress.
- People experiencing substance misuse.
- People experiencing restrictions to their limitations.
- Those with mental health issues, new or long term.
- Confusion, either new or of longer standing, e.g. delirium, dementia, hypoxia.
- Your own emotions, time pressures and other factors that may affect your behaviour (Sookoo 2018).

Professional Approach

- Ensure that you are appropriately trained in de-escalation skills and feel both confident and competent to engage in communication.
- If the situation escalates it could be that you are unintentionally aggravating the situation. In this instance you should delegate the conversation to prevent further escalation; not doing so is unprofessional and puts you and the patient at risk.
- Be aware of your scope of practice and rights: all nursing staff and all those considered emergency workers – i.e. those working in the emergency department and urgent care centres, as well as paramedics – are protected under the Assault on Emergency Workers [Offenses] Act 2018 c.23.

Equipment

- Equipment is not specifically required but be mindful that a uniform could escalate, or calm, the situation.
- Ensure that you have enough time to engage.
- Ensure that you have a way to call for help, i.e. a panic alarm, personal alarm.

Procedure

- Inform colleagues prior to approach.
- Be calm, confident and non-threatening to support early rapport (Figure 5.2).
- Listen to the patient and assess verbal and non-verbal cues that could inform your decision regarding which de-escalation strategy to use.
- Use active listening to identify the patient's concerns.
- Following initial assessment, suggest a quieter area if it is safe to do.
- Use your fundamental communication skills, and ensure that you speak slowly and calmly using VAPER (volume, articulation, pitch, emphasis and rate; Nelson-Jones 2014) to ensure that you communicate in a calm and caring manner.
- Maintain an open, non-threatening posture and encourage the patient to sit if currently standing, then ensure you follow SOLER (see Table 4.3; Egan 2014).
- Adjust your body language to ensure that you are expressing concern and support for the patient (Figure 5.3).
- Maintain appropriate social physical distancing; closeness could aggravate the aggression.
- Engage in shared ownership of the problem and work towards attaining a solution together.
- Once a solution has been found, reiterate your actions and the dates and times you will provide the patient with this information.
- If a solution is not found, continue to monitor cues whilst attempting to gain a resolution.
- If the patient then moves from early warning signs to danger signs of risk (Table 5.1), remove yourself from the situation and involve colleagues as appropriate.[1]

Red Flag

- ☛ Sudden change in consciousness level should be escalated immediately.
- ☛ If you perceive changes in behaviour to be threatening, remove yourself immediately.

References

Egan, G. (2014). *The Skilled Helper: A Problem Management and Opportunity Development Approach to Helping*, 10e. California: Brooks-Cole.

Emergency Workers (Offenses) Act 2018 c.23. https://www.legislation.gov.uk/ukpga/2018/23/contents/enacted/data.htm (accessed 17 May 2021).

National Institute for Health and Care Excellence (2015). *(NG10) Violence and Aggression: Short-Term Management in Mental Health, Health and Community Settings*. London: National Institute for Health and Care Excellence.

Nelson-Jones, R. (2014). *Nelson-Jones' Theory and Practice of Counselling and Psychotherapy*, 6e. London: Sage Publications.

Nursing & Midwifery Council (2018). *Professional Standards and Practice of Behaviour for Nurse, Midwives and Nursing Associates*. London: Nursing & Midwifery Council.

Sookoo, S. (2018). Identifying and managing risk of aggression and violence. In: *The Art and Science of Mental Health Nursing: Principles and Practice*, 4e (eds. I. Norman and I. Ryrie), 222–238. London: Open University Press.

---

1 It may be that you feel it is outside of your skillset to reach a resolution. In this instance you may want to hand over care to a more experienced colleague. You may also find yourself in a situation where you feel risk is imminent. In this instance, extract yourself and call for help. This may involve using a silent panic button.

6 Communication – difficult conversations

Background

Working effectively in healthcare requires handling a wide range of conversations daily. Most people accessing the health services are experiencing stress and anxiety that come from uncertainty and loss. It is not always clear what will become a difficult conversation and, conversely, what will turn out to be easier to talk about than we would have expected.

Fear of the unknown regarding how a conversation might go is often the key factor that results in healthcare professionals avoiding initiating conversations they feel might be difficult. Preparing yourself and attentively listening can help you to approach and navigate these conversations.

Professional Approach: Preparing Your Self

Preparing for having these conversations is of fundamental importance. Ensure you are prepared for them to happen as a normal part of daily practice, observe others, and, as with any difficult skills, take the opportunity to practise whenever you can.

Engaging in healthcare communication is hard emotional work. Recognising this and understanding the need to develop ways of managing the emotion this causes are important. Suggestions include self-care, developing relational skills, maintaining an empathic presence, taking a team approach, and retaining a professional identity (Luff et al. 2016).

Influencing Factors: What Conversations Might Be Considered Difficult?

- Cancelled treatments.
- Communicating with relatives.
- Complex health promotion discussions.
- Conversations around costs.
- Life-changing diagnosis.
- Lost belongings.
- Managing cultural differences.
- Unexpected deterioration.
- End-of-life conversations.

Influencing Factors: Requisite Qualities and Skills

1 The ability to listen.
2 A compassionate approach.
3 The courage to start or engage with conversation that maybe difficult.
4 The skills to manage a conversation that may involve a range of emotions.
5 An ability to be comfortable with silence.

Procedure: Breaking Bad News

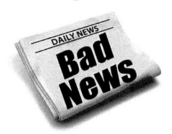

In healthcare education we often talk about the need for "breaking bad news training". It is important to be cautious with regard to making assumptions about what is bad news for another person. Sometimes a diagnosis can be a relief after months of uncertainty and symptoms. Sometimes the person has known for a while and it is a relief to be able to talk about it with someone else. Approaching these conversations can still create anxiety, however, hence the term "difficult conversations".

Hence a valuable rule is: Before you tell, ask (Bryan 2007).

Procedure: Be PREPARED

All conversations we have in healthcare are about communicating between two or more people, one of them being you. Thinking carefully about who those people are and what their experiences have been on that day before you have that conversation is an important starting point. Clayton et al. (2007) offer this useful model as we learn how to approach situations that we feel may be difficult.

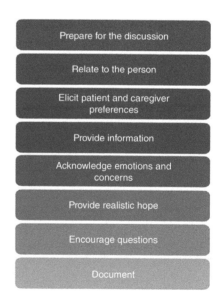

Prepare for the discussion

Relate to the person

Elicit patient and caregiver preferences

Provide information

Acknowledge emotions and concerns

Provide realistic hope

Encourage questions

Document

Procedure: Balancing Hope and Realism

Discussing difficult things can and will cause an emotional response to all who are involved. Emotional release can be cathartic; it is okay if someone cries. Learn to use tissues and empathetic silence.

People need time to process emotions. If you can give them time, they can develop new hope by refocusing on what is important to them. This happens better in an environment where people feel they can trust their healthcare professionals to take an individual-centred approach to communication (Campbell et al. 2010).

References

Bryan, L. (2007). Should ward nurses hide death from other patients. *End of Life Care* 1 (1): 79–86.

Campbell, T.C., Carey, E.C., Jackson, V.A. et al. (2010). Discussing prognosis: balancing hope and realism. *The Cancer Journal* 16 (5): 461–466.

Clayton, J.M., Hancock, K.M., Butow, P.N. et al. (2007). Clinical practice guidelines for communicating prognosis and end-of-life issues with adults in the advanced stages of a life-limiting illness, and their caregivers. *The Medical Journal of Australia* 186 (12): S77–S108.

Luff, D., Martin, E.B. Jr., Mills, K. et al. (2016). Clinicians' strategies for managing their emotions during difficult healthcare conversations. *Patient Education and Counseling* 99 (9): 1461–1466.

7 Informed consent

Figure 7.1   Implied consent.

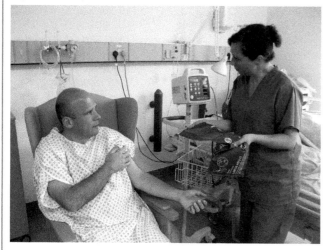

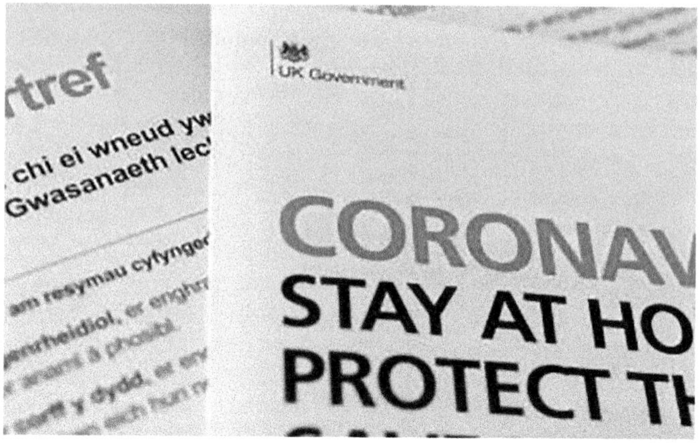

Figure 7.2   Translation material.

UK Government

...rtref
...chi ei wneud yw...
Gwasanaeth lec...

...am resymau cyfynged...
...nrheidiol, er enghr...
...enant â phosibl.
...saff y dydd, ei en...
...each hun m...

CORONAV
STAY AT HO
PROTECT TH

Figure 7.3   Materials in Braille.

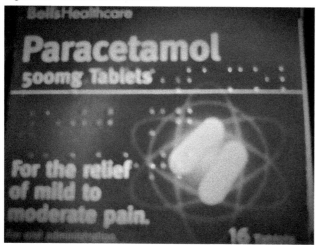

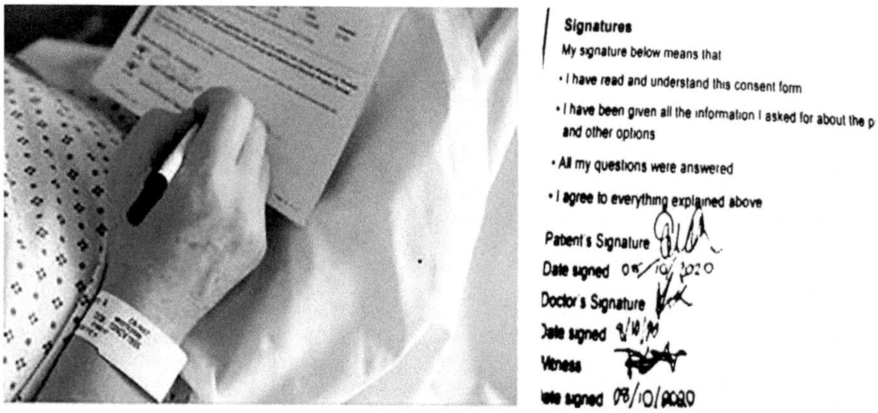

Figure 7.4   Written consent with signature.

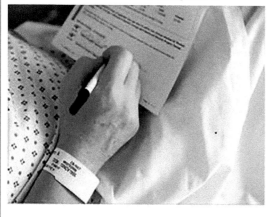

Signatures

My signature below means that

• I have read and understand this consent form

• I have been given all the information I asked for about the p
and other options

• All my questions were answered

• I agree to everything explained above

Patient's Signature

Date signed 0 /10/2020

Doctor's Signature

Date signed /10/

Witness

ate signed 08/10/2020

Clinical Nursing Skills at a Glance, First Edition. Edited by Sarah Curr and Carol Fordham-Clarke.
© 2022 John Wiley & Sons Ltd. Published 2022 by John Wiley & Sons Ltd.
Companion website: www.wiley.com/go/clinicalnursingskills

Background

- Part 4 of the Nursing & Midwifery Council (NMC) code highlights the need for informed consent to be obtained – 4.1 specifically states that we must "act in the best interests of all people at all times", recognising "that we need to respect a person's right to accept or refuse treatment" (NMC 2018, p. 7).
- For a person's rights to be respected we must ensure that they have all key information in order to be able to make an informed decision about accepting or refusing treatment.
- This informed consent can then be given in written or oral form, but it can also be implied, such as when providing the arm for blood pressure measurement (Figure 7.1).
- In healthcare, informed consent must be achieved for all interventions and this includes initial and ongoing assessments, tests, treatments, and subsequent care provision.
- It is important to note that informed consent is only valid for the period of that intervention. If that interaction is repeated, consent will need to be obtained again. This is required for all healthcare interventions.

Influencing Factors

- Language barriers – these can be mitigated by using translated material and translation services (Figure 7.2).
- Visual impairment – ensure that the patient has all usual visual aids and consider whether larger text may be available for written material. Written material is also available in braille (Figure 7.3).
- Aural impairment – ensure that the patient has all hearing aids and that these are working effectively. Consider whether a quieter area would be more appropriate to provide the information. The patient's wish for privacy and dignity must also be taken into consideration here.
- Inability to communicate – there are multiple communication tools available and patients will often have their own, so most communication challenges can be overcome. In the case of an unconscious patient, consent cannot be obtained and healthcare professionals are required to act in the best interests of the patient.
- Lack of capacity – if a lack of capacity is suspected this must then be tested.[1]

Professional Approach

- The healthcare professional who is gaining consent must ensure that they understand the information being given, are able to answer relevant questions on the topic (Royal College of Nursing 2017), and have time to undertake the task.
- To ensure informed consent, the healthcare professional must provide all key information, answer questions, and then ascertain understanding by asking questions to ensure that the information has been retained and recalled.

---

1 The healthcare professional must ascertain that the person has an impairment, which means that they cannot do one or more of the following: (i) understand information presented; (ii) retain information sufficiently to make a decision; (iii) weigh up the information provided; (iv) communicate their decision (Mental Capacity Act 2005).

- Consent must be gained voluntarily from the patient. If the patient is influenced by other healthcare professionals, family, friends, or significant others, it is our duty to report this to the multidisciplinary team caring for the patient.
- Remember that, although informed consent is a professional requirement, it is also a legal requirement. Withholding key information which then results in harm can result in a claim of negligence by omission (*Montgomery v. Lanarkshire Health Board* 2015).

Equipment

- Ensure that you have all relevant material, i.e. written material, translator service.
- Ensure you have an appropriate space to gain the consent.

Procedure – Informed Consent

- Introduce yourself and advise that you are gaining consent for the required procedure. For many procedures, you explain the procedure you are doing and ask if they consent to this. The detail required will depend on the complexity and risks of the procedure: e.g. surgery requires detailed information to be provided and written consent.
- Confirm the patient's name, date of birth, and other identifiers as required by local Trust policy.
- Explain the nature of the procedure.
- Explain why the procedure is being proposed.
- Highlight the risks of the procedure.
- Provide information on the benefits.
- Advise what will happen if the procedure is not performed, and what the prognosis will be.
- Avoid using medical jargon and check for understanding after each stage of the process.
- Provide the patient with adequate time to absorb the information given and read all written material.
- Return to obtain informed written consent, with a signature (Figure 7.4), and file this appropriately within the patient's notes.

Red Flag

- Using a family member to translate could result in the full information not being provided to the patient. This would not be valid consent and the healthcare professional could be held to account in the event of an adverse outcome.
- Do not assume that there is a lack of capacity because you feel that the decision is unwise. This could result in charges of battery (Dimond 2015).

References

Dimond, B. (2015). *Legal Aspects of Nursing*, 7e. Harlow: Pearson.

Mental Capacity Act 2005 (c.9). https://www.legislation.gov.uk/ukpga/2005/9/contents

Montgomery v. Lanarkshire Health Board (2015) UKSC 11. https://www.supremecourt.uk/cases/docs/uksc-2013-0136-judgment.pdf

Nursing & Midwifery Council (2018). *Professional Standards and Practice of Behaviour for Nurse, Midwives and Nursing Associates.* London: Nursing & Midwifery Council.

Royal College of Nursing (2017). *Principles of Consent: Guidance for Nursing Staff.* London: Royal College of Nursing.

8 Privacy and dignity

Table 8.1 Specific laws that relate to reportable activities.

Act of Parliament	Year of publication
Misuse of Drugs Act	1971
The Public Health (Control of Disease) Act	1984
Road Traffic Accident Act	2010
Terrorism Prevention and Investigation Measures Act	2011
Data Protection Act	2018

Table 8.2 Human rights articles relating to healthcare.

Article	Related to healthcare
Article 3	Freedom from torture and inhuman or degrading treatment
Article 5	Right to liberty and security
Article 8	Respect for your privacy and family life, home, and correspondence

Figure 8.1 Engaged clip for curtains.

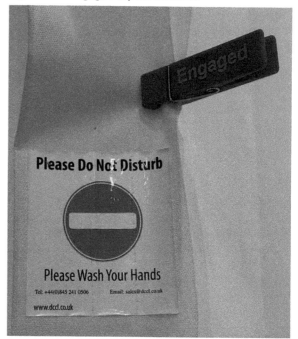

Table 8.3 The six Ps of social media.

Professionalism	Ensure professional profile and professionalism with all posted material
Positive	Keep posts positive. Grievances have no place in social media
Patient/person	Think about the person. If this post concerned you, would you want it to be uploaded to social media?
Protect	Protect yourself, your colleagues, employer, and the public
Pause	Stop and think. If unsure do not post

Source: Nursing & Midwifery Council (2018b).

Clinical Nursing Skills at a Glance, First Edition. Edited by Sarah Curr and Carol Fordham-Clarke.
© 2022 John Wiley & Sons Ltd. Published 2022 by John Wiley & Sons Ltd.
Companion website: www.wiley.com/go/clinicalnursingskills

Background

- The Nursing & Midwifery Council (NMC) code, section 5, focuses on prioritising people, which highlights upholding dignity whilst also focusing on respecting people's right to privacy and confidentiality (NMC 2018a).
- Privacy falls under confidentiality in law, which focuses on handling data appropriately and securely, and only sharing it for specific reasons (Data Protection Act 2018).
- Under law, confidentiality can be waived in order to prevent harm to oneself, by self or others, and to prevent harm to others. Specific laws refer to activities that require referral to authority bodies (Table 8.1).
- Supporting privacy and dignity is also a human right with three specific articles of the UK Humans Rights Act (1998) focusing on these (Table. 8.2).
- Privacy and dignity also refer to maintaining the privacy and dignity of patients, employers, and other employees actions outside of the work environment – this is specifically important when engaging with social media.

Influencing Factors

- Emergency situations – when saving life is a priority, both privacy and dignity can be forgotten. Closing the curtain or door can be helpful, but as multiple members of the team may be entering and leaving the room, closing the curtain or door of surrounding patients can reduce exposure.
- The unconscious patient is unable to express preferences – this information may be provided by other sources (e.g. family members, patient's notes) but advocating for the patient is also required in these circumstances.
- Lack of capacity – sharing of information in these situations can be challenging. Avoid assuming that information can be provided and look for a lasting power of attorney form.

Professional Approach

- Time pressures – these pressures can result in a lack of privacy when providing sensitive care.
- Time pressures – these pressures can also cause healthcare workers to disregard patient dignity by not considering patients' preferences. which could be based on cultural, religious or other practices.
- Maintaining privacy requires healthcare professionals to treat the patient as an individual for each individual interaction; not doing so can disregard legal and professional requirements.

Equipment

- A 'do not disturb' clip to use with curtains (Figure 8.1).
- A roller blind for door windows.
- Appropriate documentation security.

Procedure – Key Considerations

- Ensure the procedure is fully explained and informed consent is obtained.
- Check that there will be no interruptions for the duration of the procedure; use 'do not disturb' signs.

- Advise members of your team, and the nurse in charge where you will be, as appropriate.
- Ask the patient their preference for the procedure, e.g. "Would you prefer for the curtain to be open or closed while I measure your vital signs?"
- Explain what you are doing throughout.
- Ensure the patient has adequate levels of privacy for their requirements before you leave the area.
- Follow the record-keeping guidance for clear, accurate, professional documentation.
- Follow data protection requirements for storage of all patient data (Data Protection Act 2018).
- Note – supporting the patient to be independent when providing person care is preferred but not always possible. Encouraging the patient to provide care for their genitalia can support privacy and maintain dignity.

Procedure – Social Media

Unprofessional and unlawful conduct across social media has resulted in professional bodies providing guidance on managing your social media profile (GMC 2013; NMC 2018b). The NMC has recommended that professionals follow the six Ps before posting on any platform (see Table 8.3). It has also highlighted that fitness to practise will be questioned in the following instances:

- There is sharing of confidential information inappropriately, i.e. without patient consent or providing employer – and thus healthcare provider – details.
- There is posting of unprofessional comments about people they provide care for, other team members, and/or employer.
- There is posting that could be considered as bullying or exploitation of patients, other team members, and/or the employing organisation.
- There is posting of pictures or videos without the party's consent (NMC 2018b).

Red Flag

- ☛ Failing to comply with professional requirements can result in a fitness-to-practice review and lead to removal from the professional register.
- ☛ Failure to follow the law will bring legal recriminations, which could include tribunal cases brought by an employer, breach of professional negligence under case law, or a breach of a specific Act of Parliament. These incur penalties such as fines, community sentencing, and imprisonment.

References

Data Protection Act (2018) c12. www.legislation.gov.uk/ukpga/2018/12/contents/enacted (accessed 22 April 2020).

General Medical Council (2013). *Doctor's Use of Social Media*. London: General Medical Council.

Human Rights Act (1998) c.42. www.legislation.gov.uk/ukpga/1998/42/contents (accessed 22 April 2020).

Nursing & Midwifery Council (2018a). *Professional Standards and Practice of Behaviour for Nurse, Midwives and Nursing Associates*. London: Nursing & Midwifery Council.

Nursing & Midwifery Council (2018b). *Guidance on Using Social Media Responsibly*. London: Nursing & Midwifery Council.

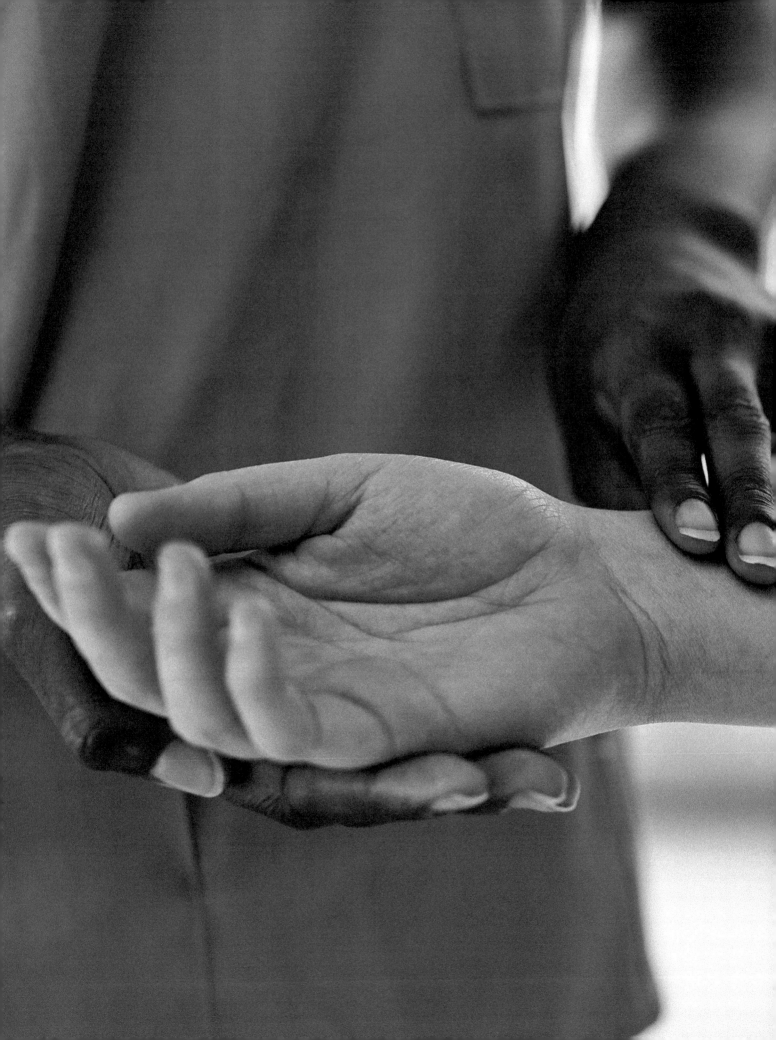

Mandatory skills

Part 3

Chapters

9 Moving and handling

Figure 9.1   Sit to stand.

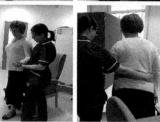
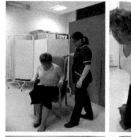
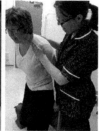

Figure 9.2   Walking with assistance of one.

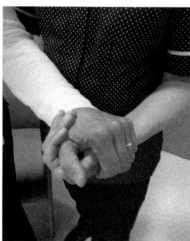

Figure 9.3   Walking with assistance of two.

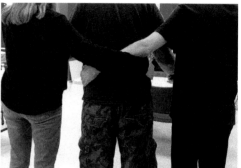

Figure 9.4   Walking with a frame.

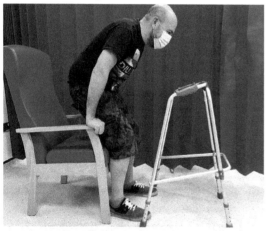
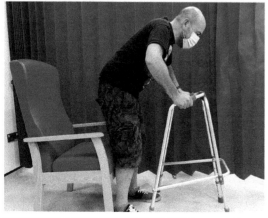

Table 9.1 Using TILEO for safety in manual handling.

Task	Does the task include twisting, stooping, bending, pushing, pulling, or sudden movement?
Individual	Consider the patient and the handler with respect to health, e.g. disability, pregnancy
Load	Consider weight, stability, ability to grip
Environment	Consider space constraints, flooring – stable, same level, hot/cold conditions
Other factors	Is the movement hindered by infusions, traction, drains? Have you the correct working equipment?

Source: Based on Smith 2011.

Figure 9.5   Standing to sitting.

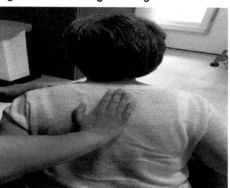

Clinical Nursing Skills at a Glance, First Edition. Edited by Sarah Curr and Carol Fordham-Clarke.
© 2022 John Wiley & Sons Ltd. Published 2022 by John Wiley & Sons Ltd.
Companion website: www.wiley.com/go/clinicalnursingskills

Background

- Moving and handling (MH) refers to the assistance given to a load[1] to enable it to move.
- These include lifting, putting down, pulling, pushing, carrying, supporting a load whilst static, throwing or moving by hand or bodily force.
- MH is governed by the Health and Safety at Work Act 1974 and welfare legislation (National Back Exchange 2010), which include regulations for employers and employees to understand, and subsequently follow, to ensure their own and others' safety.
- MH procedures are often utilised in healthcare settings when assisting a patient with their mobility but can be applied to any environment where the MH of a load is required, e.g. supermarkets, warehouses, and mechanics' garages.
- MH is often required to maintain the safety of the patient but in undertaking these procedures healthcare providers need to ensure their own safety.
- Back and musculoskeletal injuries are one of the most common causes of sick leave among healthcare professionals (HSE 2015). These are often a result of poor MH techniques.

Influencing Factors

- Mobility and assistance requirements can change daily and thus a discussion with the patient on how much they feel able to do is required before supporting with any activity.
- Changes in ability to mobilise should be documented when they occur. It could be that the patient has become more unwell, has increased pain, or requires bed rest post-procedure.

Procedure – Key Points to Remember

Avoid

- Performing any MH procedures.
- Can the patient move themselves with direction?
- Is there equipment that can be used?

Assess and Plan

- It is essential to assess and plan before any MH procedures.
- The acronym TILEO (task, individual, load, environment, other) can be used (Table 9.1; Smith 2011).

Spine in Line

Keep the spine's natural position to reduce any injury or damage while providing ease of movement.

Load Close

Keep the load close to your body as this reduces pressure on the lower back and provides ease of movement.

Stable Base, Soft knees

Provides ease of movement in a safe way.

Centre of Gravity

Should be neutral for safety.

Professional Approach

- Obtain informed consent.
- Provide reassurance.
- Ensure effective teamwork and communication between all involved, including the patient.

---

1 A load refers to a person or any object.

- Maintain privacy and dignity.
- Work within your sphere of competence.

Moving and Handling Techniques

The following techniques are commonly used in healthcare settings when a person requires assistance with mobility. The techniques vary from minimal assistance to full assistance with the aid of MH equipment.

Sit to Stand

- This method can be used when assisting a patient from a sitting to a standing position if safe, independent, mobilisation is not possible (Figure 9.1).
- Before starting the process, establish if the person will be able to stand. For a patient to be able to stand, they need good core muscles as well as strength in their arms and legs.

Walking with Assistance of One

- Once the person is standing, stand slightly behind but close to the person requiring assistance. Walk with your hands in a palm-to-palm hold (Figure 9.2).
- Ask the patient to look in the direction they are wanting to walk in and let them initiate the first step.
- Walk with the patient and provide reassurance.

Walking with Assistance of Two

- Follow the above steps, with the second handler doing the same on the patient's other side.
- Ensure both handlers' arms cross over, across the back of the patient, to provide further support (Figure 9.3).

Walking with a Frame

- Inform the patient that once they are standing the frame will be placed within reach.
- The patient's hands should be placed either side of the frame for support while they walk.
- The frame should be moved first, followed by the patient's feet (Figure 9.4).

Standing to Sitting

- Ensure the back of the patient's legs are touching the chair.
- The patient reaches for the chair behind them with bottom out towards the chair to sit.
- Your hand can come to the middle of their back and apply gentle pressure to guide the patient back into the chair (Figure 9.5).

Red Flags

- Never use a frame to assist standing.
- Do not walk too close to the patient's hips; allow for natural sway and movement of hips.
- Changes in mobility, particularly any weakness, should be noted and escalated as appropriate.

References

Health and Safety Executive (HSE) (2015) *Health and Safety in the Health and Social Care Sector in Great Britain, 2014/15*. www.hse.gov.uk/statistics/industry/healthservices/health.

Smith, J. (2011). *The Guide to the Handling of People*, 6e. London: National Back Pain Association.

The National Back Exchange (2010). *Guidelines for Manual Handling*, 3e. Towcester: The National Back Exchange.

10 Moving and handling: turning in bed, transfers, and hoisting

Figure 10.1 Turning in bed – two-person.

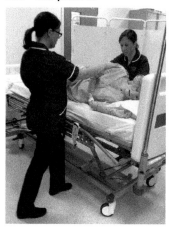

Figure 10.2 Preparing the slide sheet.

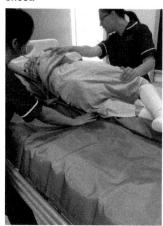

Figure 10.3 Using the slide sheet.

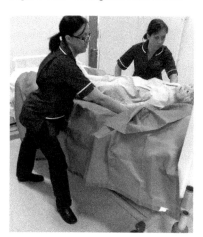

Figure 10.4 Lateral transfer.

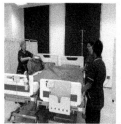 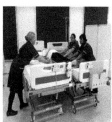

Figure 10.5 Using a hoist.

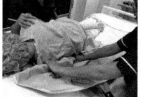 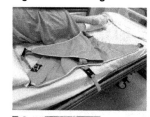 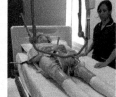

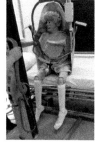 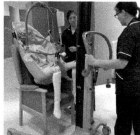 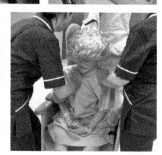

Clinical Nursing Skills at a Glance, First Edition. Edited by Sarah Curr and Carol Fordham-Clarke.
© 2022 John Wiley & Sons Ltd. Published 2022 by John Wiley & Sons Ltd.
Companion website: www.wiley.com/go/clinicalnursingskills

Background

Some patients can require further assistance with their mobility and equipment may be required. An assessment using TILEO (task, individual, load, environment, other factors Table 9.1; Smith 2011) as well as the key procedural points, outlined in Chapter 9, must be considered before undertaking the task. This includes raising the bed to the correct height for those performing the skill.

Influencing Factors

- Always ensure that there is enough time to complete the task – both for staff and the patient.
- Consider each individual person who requires support and consider how many people will be required before undertaking the task.
- Consider if analgesia is required before supporting the patient to move position.

Professional Approach

- Ensure informed consent is obtained.
- Maintain privacy and dignity.
- Effective communication and teamwork are vital during these procedures.
- Provide reassurance and, where possible, involve the patient.
- All individuals should work within their sphere of competence for the safety of all involved.

Equipment

Depending on the procedure you will require:

- The appropriate number of competent personnel.
- Sliding sheet/s.
- Correctly sized hoist sling.
- Hoist.

Procedure – Turn in Bed

This method can be undertaken with the patient and one handler only if the patient is able to partially move and aid themselves in turning onto their side. If the patient is unable to move at all then two handlers will be required.

- Ask, or assist, the patient to bend the leg furthest away from you, position with the foot flat on the bed.
- If required, assist the patient in rolling towards you by placing one hand on the hip and the other on the shoulder and then turn (Figure 10.1).

Procedure – Moving in Bed Using a Slide Sheet

This enables a patient to be moved up and down and from side to side in a bed. It requires a minimum of two people and should not be attempted if only one trained individual is available. **NB**: Attach two slide sheets to ensure less friction when moving the patient.

- To start, turn the patient on their side.
- Roll the two slide sheets together halfway and place alongside the patient's body (Figure 10.2).
- Turn the patient onto their other side over the rolled slide sheets and then pull the sheets out flat.
- The patient can then return to lying on their back with the slide sheets flat underneath them.
- Facing the head of the bed, the trained individuals adopt a stable position, feet apart, and hold the slide sheet (Figure 10.3).
- The patient is then moved as the trained individuals transfer body weight from the back to the front foot.
- This is coordinated by using the command "ready, steady, slide".

Procedure – Lateral Transfers

- This enables a patient to be moved in a lateral position.
- This transfer is often used when it is necessary to move a person from one bed to another, i.e. when you are transferring between wards and using a transfer board.
- With the patient on their side and a sliding sheet flat underneath, insert the transfer board under the slide sheet, ensuring that the patient's head is on the board.
- Roll the patient into the supine position. Half of the board should be on the bed and the other half hanging in mid-air until the other bed is moved into position (Figure 10.4).
- Ensure there are enough trained individuals.
- The trained individuals stand in a stable position, two to push and two to pull on the command of "ready, steady, slide".

Procedure – Hoisting

- A hoist is a piece of equipment used to move people from one place to another when they are unable to move in any other way.
- A hoist can be used to hoist from a bed to a wheelchair, a chair, a commode, another bed, a trolley or from the floor.
- There are many hoist types with slings that can only be used with the hoist for which they are designed.
- Most manufactured slings are for single patient use, for infection control, and there are specially designed ones for use in water should you require to hoist a person into a bath.
- Using a hoist always requires a minimum of two trained individuals.

   NB: It is important to familiarise yourself with the type of hoist and slings available to use in your clinical area.

   The following checks must be carried out before a hoist is used:

- Ensure there is a recent safety certificate.
- Ensure the manual winding-down function works.
- Ensure that all electronic functions work.
- Ensure that there is a battery check.
- Ensure that there is a brake check.
- Ensure the weight that the hoist can support is suitable for the load you are lifting.
- Ensure the sling is measured against the patient being hoisted for correct sizing. Measure from the top of the head to the base of the spine, from hip to knee, and finally from shoulder to shoulder. Together these give you the correct size of sling for that patient. Each sling manufacturer will give you specific sling measurements.
- Figure 10.5 shows how a patient is hoisted from a bed to a chair. The same principles and procedures can be applied for other hoist transfers.

Red Flags

- ➤ Ensure the bed brakes are on for sliding sheet transfers.
- ➤ The brakes must never be on when using the hoist.
- ➤ Never leave patients in a hoist for extended periods.
- ➤ The sling must always be removed from under the patient when not required to prevent pressure sores.
- ➤ Always use the required number of trained individuals.
- ➤ Never use bed sheets as sliding sheets.

References

Smith, J. (2011). *The Guide to the Handling of People*, 6e. London: Back Care: National Back Pain Association.

11 Basic life support

Figure 11.1   Head tilt/chin lift.

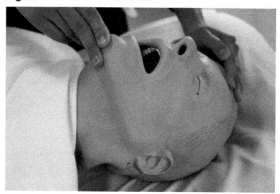

Figure 11.2   Chest compressions.

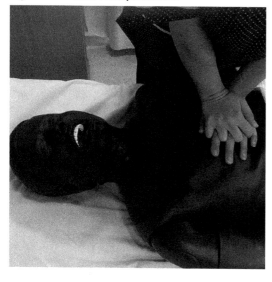

Figure 11.3   Mouth-to-mouth resuscitation.

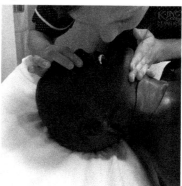

Figure 11.4   Defibrillator pad placement.

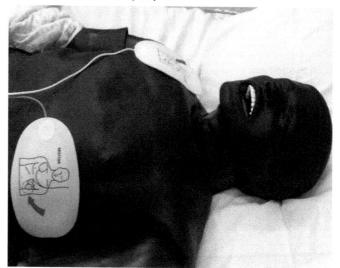

Clinical Nursing Skills at a Glance, First Edition. Edited by Sarah Curr and Carol Fordham-Clarke.
© 2022 John Wiley & Sons Ltd. Published 2022 by John Wiley & Sons Ltd.
Companion website: www.wiley.com/go/clinicalnursingskills

Background

Adult Basic Life Support (BLS) aims to keep the airway open and support breathing while maintaining circulation through cardio-pulmonary resuscitation (CPR). The heart is the body's pump that moves blood around the circulatory system. As the transport of blood, and thus oxygen and nutrients, is essential to life, CPR is used to get this oxygenated blood to the vital organs when the heart has stopped pumping. As it is the respiratory system that brings oxygen from the air into our lungs, it is also necessary to provide the patient with oxygen during this process. In BLS, this is done through rescue breaths, as outlined below.

NB: The European Resuscitation Council guide our performance of this skill. The key guidelines are from Monsieurs et al. (2015) with an update from the Resuscitation Council UK (2021).

Influencing Factors – Chain of Survival

Although BLS is important there are four key factors that the European Resuscitation Council (Monsieurs et al. 2015) recognise as factors improving patient outcome:

- Early recognition and call for help.
- Early CPR.
- Early defibrillation.
- Post-resuscitation care.

Professional Approach

When undertaking BLS it is important to work within your own level of competence and consider the patient's privacy and dignity (Nursing & Midwifery Council 2018). Consider the following:

- Do all personnel need to be present?
- Is it possible to shield the patient from all but necessary caregivers?

Procedure – Basic Life Support

When attending to a collapsed individual, the **DRAB** mnemonic (Monsieurs et al. 2015) can be followed. Assess for:

- **Danger** – consider the collapsed individual, bystanders, yourself.
- **Response** – check for response, speak to the individual. If no response shake the shoulders.

If the person responds, leave in the current position, attempt to establish what is wrong, and then go for help. If there is no response shout or call for help immediately. Then:

- **Airway** – open airway by performing head tilt and chin lift, with one hand on the forehead tilting the head back and the finger-tips of your other hand under the chin to lift the chin (Figure 11.1).
- **Breathing** – at this stage:
  - *Look* – for movement of the chest.
  - *Listen* – at patient's mouth for breath sounds.
  - *Feel* – for air against your cheek.
  NB: This should be for no more than 10 seconds.

Note that if SARS-COV-2 or any other potentially lethal respiratory infection is suspected, full personal protective equipment for an aerosol-generating procedure is required before commencing BLS which commences with CPR (Resuscitation Council UK 2020).

If after these interventions the person is breathing normally, place into the recovery position. If not call 999 (in the UK), or ask a fellow bystander to, and commence CPR:

- Kneel by the collapsed individual and place the heel of your hand on the patient's chest.
- Place the heel of the other hand on top of the first hand and interlock your fingers.

- Position yourself vertically above the patient's chest and compress the chest to 5–6 cm at a rate of 100–120/minute; do this 30 times (Figure 11.2).

After 30 compressions perform two rescue breaths if trained to do so:

- Open airway again using head tilt/chin lift.
- Pinch the soft part of the patient's nose to close it using the index finger and thumb of the hand on the forehead.
- Take a normal breath, place a seal around the patient's mouth and breathe steadily, over one second, into the patient's mouth while simultaneously watching the chest rise (Figure 11.3).
- Do one further breathe and re-commence CPR.
- If rescue breaths do not make the chest rise at the next ventilation attempt, check the patient's mouth for obstruction.
- Continue until the patient shows signs of regaining consciousness, help arrives, or you become exhausted.
- If there is more than one person in attendance, the person delivering CPR should be changed every two minutes to prevent exhaustion.

NB: Only give rescue breaths if trained to do so.

Procedure – Automated External Defibrillators

Resuscitation Council guidelines (Monsieurs et al. 2015) highlight the importance of early defibrillation. Automated external defibrillators (AEDs) can be used both in and out of hospital settings:

- Ensure that you follow the adult BLS guideline and request an AED once the patient is recognised as unresponsive and not breathing, if there is more than one person in attendance.
- Once the AED arrives switch on and place the electrode pads on the patient's chest in the correct position (Figure 11.4).
- Continue CPR during attachment and then follow AED spoken or visual instructions.

Signs of Regaining Consciousness

- Coughing.
- Opening eyes.
- Moving purposefully.
- Breathing normally.

Red Flags

- Agonal breathing is irregular, gasping, laboured breathing and is not normal. If present, start CPR immediately.
- Consider your own safety when undertaking CPR.
- You can consider using mouth-to-nose ventilation if the patient's mouth is seriously injured.
- Do not use mouth-to-mouth or a pocket mask for respiratory conditions, such as SARS-COV-2, to prevent transmission of infection.

References

Monsieurs, K.G., Nolan, J.P., Bossaert, L.L. et al. (2015). European Resuscitation Council guidelines for resuscitation 2015 section 1. Executive summary. *Resuscitation* 95: 1–80.

Nursing & Midwifery Council (2018). *Professional Standards of Practice and Behaviour for Nurses, Midwives and Nursing Associates*. London: Nursing and Midwifery Council.

Resuscitation Council UK (2020). *Guidance for the Resuscitation of Adult COVID-19 Patients in Acute Hospital Settings*. London: Resuscitation Council UK.

Resuscitation Council UK (2021). *Adult basic life support Guidelines*. Available from https://www.resus.org.uk/library/2021-resuscitation-guidelines/adult-basic-life-support-guidelines

12 The choking patient; the recovery position

Figure 12.1   Back slap.

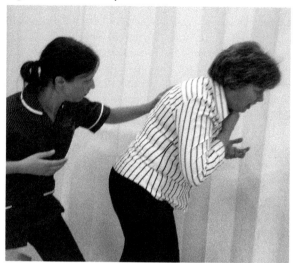

Figure 12.2   Abdominal thrusts.

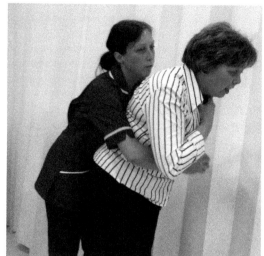

Figure 12.3   Recovery position.

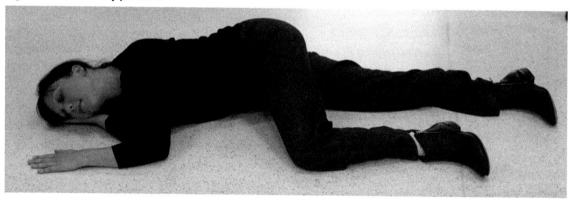

Clinical Nursing Skills at a Glance, First Edition. Edited by Sarah Curr and Carol Fordham-Clarke.
© 2022 John Wiley & Sons Ltd. Published 2022 by John Wiley & Sons Ltd.
Companion website: www.wiley.com/go/clinicalnursingskills

Background

Obstructions to the airway can be categorised as upper or lower airway obstructions. Airway obstruction is recognised as a life-threatening condition, as obstruction to the airway can prevent movement of the respiratory gases, both in and out. Choking is an upper airway obstruction and can be caused by swallowing or inhaling a foreign body, resulting in a mild or severe obstruction. In order to resolve this obstruction, the foreign body needs to be dislodged and removed.

NB: Remember if any interventions are used, the patient must be taken to hospital for further assessment.

Professional Approach

- Reassure the patient and explain what you are doing: informed consent can be obtained through verbal and non-verbal communication.
- Remember the patient's privacy and dignity and protect these as much as possible.

NB: Remember that bystanders can become useful members of your team. Even if symptoms resolve, the patient will require medical attention and a full assessment.

Procedure – Choking Assessment

It is essential to ascertain if the person is choking. The conscious patient can be asked if they are choking. If the patient can answer in the affirmation, they can:

- Speak.
- Cough.
- Breathe.

This can be recognised as **mild** choking and they should be encouraged to cough.

If the patient is unable to answer through speech they may nod. This can be classified as **severe** choking and they may experience:

- Difficulty in breathing.
- Wheezy breath sounds.
- Silent cough attempts.
- Unconsciousness.

If the choking is severe, active management is required. This involves up to five back slaps, fewer if it resolves, and up to five abdominal thrusts.

Procedure – Back Slaps (5)

These are commenced once severe choking is recognised:

- Stand to the side and slightly behind the patient.
- Place one hand on the chest to support and lean patient forward.
- Deliver one back slap between the shoulder blades.
- Check to see if airway obstruction is resolved. If not commence a further four, checking after each back slap is delivered (Figure 12.1).

Procedure – Abdominal Thrusts (5)

Abdominal thrusts, previously called the Heimlich manoeuvre, are commenced if choking is unresolved after five back slaps:

- Stand behind the patient with both arms placed around the upper abdomen.
- Lean the patient forward.
- Clench your fist and place between the umbilicus and the bottom of the sternum.
- Grasp this hand with the other and pull upwards and inwards (Figure 12.2).
- Repeat a further four times or until obstruction is resolved.

NB: If the choking continues it will be necessary to alternate between 5 back slaps and 5 abdominal thrusts and call for help.

Recovery Position

The recovery position is advised in the unconscious patient with the aim of maintaining the patency of the airway when the patient may be unable to. It prevents the tongue from obstructing the airway and allows for draining of gastric content and thus prevents aspiration. The recovery position should not be used in a patient who is not breathing normally or who has an impaired circulation and is intended to put the patient in a stable position (Berg et al. 2011). The Resuscitation Council UK recommends the following sequence of actions to place an individual into the recovery position (Figure 12.3):

- Remove any glasses, if present.
- Kneel beside the patient and ensure that both legs are straight.
- Place the arm nearest to you out at right angles to the body, elbow bent with the hand palm up.
- Bring the far arm across the chest, and hold the back of the hand against the individual's cheek nearest to you.
- With your other hand, grasp the far leg just above the knee and pull it up, keeping the foot on the ground.
- Keeping the hand pressed against the cheek, pull on the far leg to roll the individual towards you and onto the side.
- Adjust the upper leg so that both the hip and knee are bent at right angles.
- Tilt the head back to make sure that the airway remains open.
- If necessary, adjust the hand under the cheek to keep the head tilted and facing downwards, thus allowing any liquid to drain from the mouth.
- Check that the patient is breathing regularly.

NB: If the recovery position must be maintained for **more than 30 minutes** ensure that you turn the patient onto the opposite side to relieve any pressure on the lower arm.

Red Flags

- Unresolved symptoms despite interventions.
- Unexplained additional symptoms, e.g. dysphasia.
- Unconsciousness; commence Basic Life Support.

References

Berg, R.A., Hemphill, R., Abella, B.S. et al. (2011). Part 5: adult basic life support 2010: American Heart Association guidelines for cardiopulmonary resuscitation and emergency cardiovascular care. *Circulation* 124 (15): e402.

13 Infection control

Figure 13.1 Chain of infection.

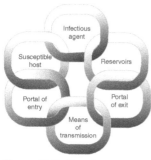

Figure 13.2 Five moments for hand hygiene. Source: Based on World Health Organization (2009).

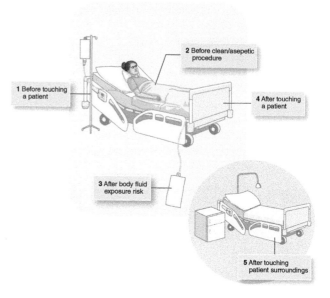

1 Before touching a patient
2 Before clean/asepetic procedure
3 After body fluid exposure risk
4 After touching a patient
5 After touching patient surroundings

Figure 13.3 Routine hand cleansing procedure.

How to wash hands correctly and reduce infection

1 Rub palm to palm
2 Rub the back of both palms
3 Rub palms again with fingers interlaced
4 Rub backs of interlaced fingers
5 Remember to wash back thumbs
6 Rub both palms with fingertips
7 Wash hands under running water using soap, rinse and do thoroughly

Figure 13.4 Clinical waste disposal in hospital.

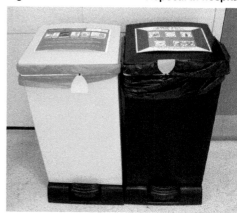

Figure 13.5 Personal protective equipment – removal.

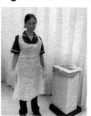 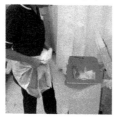

Table 13.1 Personal protective equipment.

Equipment	Use
Gloves	Non-sterile gloves must be worn for all procedures where contact with body fluids occurs Sterile gloves are worn for ANTT procedures Hands **must** be washed before and after the wearing of gloves
Aprons	Must be worn for all patient contact Must be removed and changed between activities and patients
Eye protection	Must be fit for purpose by enclosing the eye area at the top and sides (eyeglasses are **not** a substitute for clinical eye protectors) Should be worn where there is a risk of splashing of body fluids
Face masks	Surgical face masks FFP respirators should be worn by frontline staff where a patient is known/suspected to have an infection spread via the aerosol route. The FFP3 respirator must be fit-tested in order to check that an adequate seal is achieved
Sterile gowns and shoe covers	May be required when working in areas where invasive procedures are performed

ANTT, aseptic non-touch technique; FFP, filtering facepiece.

Clinical Nursing Skills at a Glance, First Edition. Edited by Sarah Curr and Carol Fordham-Clarke.
© 2022 John Wiley & Sons Ltd. Published 2022 by John Wiley & Sons Ltd.
Companion website: www.wiley.com/go/clinicalnursingskills

Background

All patients in hospital or community settings are at risk of infections. All healthcare practitioners must follow standard infection control procedures to break the chain of infection and prevent the transmission of microorganisms (Figure 13.1).

Influencing Factors

- The environment.
- Hand hygiene.
- Use of personal protective equipment (PPE).
- Appropriate waste disposal.
- Use of source isolation and protective isolation procedures.
- Aseptic non-touch techniques.

Professional Approach

Patients, significant others, and family members are more aware of the need for infection control and may seek clarification of healthcare professionals' hand hygiene procedures. They may also need support following hygiene measures when visiting. Always ensure that hand rub is readily available.

Professional Approach – Dress Code

- Healthcare workers must conform to national dress code requirements (Loveday et al. 2014).
- The healthcare provider will also require some staff to follow uniform policy.
- Dress code requirements are as follows:
  - No clothing below the elbow when in contact with patients.
  - Nails must be short, clean, and free from nail polish; false nails are prohibited.
  - No jewellery on the hands or wrists. Trusts may allow the wearing of a plain, removable wedding band.
  - Hair must be clean, tidy, away from the face and above the collar.

Procedure – Hand Hygiene

Effective hand hygiene is the most important individual infection control measure. The World Health Organization (WHO 2009) recommends that healthcare workers clean their hands according to the "5 Moments for Hand Hygiene" (see Figure 13.2). Hand hygiene incorporates handwashing with soap and water and the use of hand rubs (alcohol/chlorhexidine-based gels or foams).

Procedure – Hand Washing

- Run tap to obtain warm water.
- Wet hands.
- Apply enough soap to obtain a lather.
- Follow the systematic steps below to ensure all surfaces of the hands and wrists are adequately cleansed:
  - Vigorous rubbing motion should be employed for 20–30 seconds.
  - Rub palms together.
  - Rub the back of both hands.
  - Interlace fingers and rub together.
  - Interlock fingers and rub the back of fingers of both hands.
  - Rub both thumbs in a rotating manner.
  - Rub fingertips against palms on both hands.
  - Wash both wrists by rotational movement of the opposite hand (Figure 13.3).
- Rinse hands thoroughly under running water.
- Dry hands thoroughly using paper towels.
- Avoid contaminating hands by touching taps and other surfaces.
- Dispose of all paper towels in general waste bin using the foot pedal to open it.
- The entire handwashing procedure should take between 40 and 60 seconds.

Procedure – Use of Hand Rubs

- Hand rubs may be used as an alternative to handwashing when hands are not visibly soiled or have been in contact with body fluids.
- Follow the same procedure as for handwashing ensuring that **all surfaces** of your hands are thoroughly covered with the rub.
- Allow to dry before proceeding.
- This procedure should take 20–30 seconds.

Personal Protective Equipment

Personal protective equipment is given in Table 13.1.

Procedure – Waste Disposal

- Clinical waste must be disposed of in the appropriate containers to ensure safety for patients, visitors, and healthcare workers.
- Ensure that the appropriate clinical and non-clinical waste bin is used for disposal of waste (Figure 13.4).
- Gloves and aprons need to be removed in such a way as to contain any surface microorganisms and not contaminate the individual or the local environment. It is recommended gloves be removed before apron (Loveday et al. 2014) (Figure 13.5a,b).
- To minimise handling by laundry workers, contaminated linen should be placed in red soluble laundry bags and promptly removed from the area.

Isolation

The use of isolation prevents cross-infection between infected and non-infected areas. Isolation precautions used in the healthcare setting include:

Source isolation	Isolating an infected patient or grouping together isolated patients
Protective isolation	Isolating a vulnerable patient who is particularly susceptible to an infection, i.e. immunocompromised

- Follow Trust policy and the guidance of the infection control team when implementing isolation practices in relation to PPE, hand hygiene, and waste disposal.
- Consider the additional emotional and psychological impacts on patients who are undergoing isolation.

Red Flags

- Hand cleansing must still be performed on removing gloves.
- Alcohol gel is ineffective against some spore-producing microorganisms – therefore when caring for patients with diarrhoea or vomiting, cleanse hands with soap and water.
- Soap and water must be used when hands are visibly dirty.
- Utilising a standardised systematic approach to hand hygiene enables all surfaces of the hands and wrists to be cleansed.
- Follow infection control guidelines to protect the patient and yourself.

References

Loveday, H.P., Wilson, J.A., Pratt, R.J. et al. (2014). Epic 3: National Evidence-Based Guidelines for preventing healthcare-associated infections in NHS hospitals in England. *Journal of Hospital Infection* 86S1: S1–S70. Available at www.his.org.uk/files/3113/8693/4808/epic3_National_Evidence-Based_Guidelines_for_Preventing_HCAI_in_NHSE.pdf.

WHO (2009) *WHO Guidelines on Hand Hygiene in Health Care: First Global Patient Safety Challenge: Clean Care Is Safer Care.* Geneva: WHO. https://www.who.int/gpsc/tools/Five_moments/en/ (accessed 18 May 2021).

Medicine management

Figure 14.1 Check patient ID against prescription.

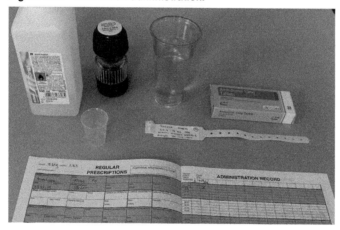

Figure 14.3 Recording medication not given.

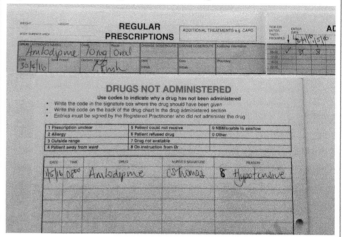

Figure 14.2 Medication administration.

Clinical Nursing Skills at a Glance, First Edition. Edited by Sarah Curr and Carol Fordham-Clarke.
© 2022 John Wiley & Sons Ltd. Published 2022 by John Wiley & Sons Ltd.
Companion website: www.wiley.com/go/clinicalnursingskills

Background

- Medication is commonly prescribed, dispensed, and administered within the healthcare setting.
- Medications can be for prophylactic use, to treat disease, to treat symptoms, for pain management, or for diagnostic purposes.
- Medicines management is a key component of care delivery, whether prescribing, administering, or dispensing.
- The Nursing & Midwifery Council (NMC) recognises that professional accountability in ensuring the safe administration of medicines is a prerequisite of the registered nurse (NMC 2018).
- The Medicines and Healthcare products Regulatory Authority (MHRA) highlights the need for medicines management to involve safe and effective use of medicines while ensuring the maximum benefit to the patient/client/service user (MHRA 2012).

Pharmacodynamics and Pharmacokinetics

- Pharmacodynamics is described as the study of how a drug affects the body and examines the biochemical and physiological actions of the drug within the body.
- As healthcare professionals, it is important to have an awareness of these effects to provide the patient with information and monitor for potential side-effects.
- Pharmacokinetics is the study of how a drug is altered within the body. This includes how it is absorbed, distributed, and eliminated.
- Healthcare professionals must consider the appropriateness of the route used for the individual patient and if there are any liver (distribution/metabolism) or renal (elimination) impairments that could potentially cause drug toxicity if dosages are not altered.
- Healthcare professionals must always have knowledge of the medication prior to administration.
- The British National Formulary (**BNF**), which is updated every six months, can be utilised as a resource for medication administration, safe prescribing, and dispensing.

Professional Approach

When giving medication, it is necessary to ensure the patient knows which medications are being administered and why. Although it is the patient's right to refuse medication, this needs to be an informed choice and as such all relevant information should be provided. If giving medication via a route that will expose the patient, the person need to be made aware of this and informed consent obtained so that privacy and dignity can be maintained.

Procedure

When administering medication, consider the nine rights (Elliot and Liu 2010):

- Right patient.
- Right dose.
- Right drug.
- Right route.
- Right time.
- Right documentation.
- Right action.
- Right form.
- Right response.

When administering medication, it is essential that the above checks have been performed, that allergy status has been checked (Figure 14.1) and that the prescriber's signature is present (Figure 14.2). It is also necessary to check for the valid period (start and finish times) of medication that requires this and check the expiry date of all drug compositions. Immediately after administration, a clear, accurate record must be made, either written on the prescription chart or recorded digitally on electronic prescriptions, and a rationale provided when medication is omitted (Figure 14.3).

NB: Student nurses only give medication under direct supervision from a registered nurse. Both parties sign off all medications given.

Controlled Drugs

The prescription and administration of controlled drugs falls under the Misuse of Drugs Act 1971. In secondary care two signatures are required and this can include a student nurse, but it is important to refer to local Trust policy. Both signatories must be assessed as competent and be involved in all stages of the process.

Classes of Medication

There are three classes of medication, described as:

- Prescription-only medication (POMs).
- Pharmacy-only medicines.
- General sales list (GSL).

Medication Supplying Methods

- Patient-specific directions (PSDs).
- Patient group directions (PGDs).

Self-administration

If a patient self-administers in the secondary care setting, the medication administration responsibility remains that of the healthcare professional overseeing the administration. The healthcare professional, usually the nurse, must undertake an ongoing assessment to ensure the patient continues to have the capacity to self-administer.

Patient-specific Medications

These are written instructions from a registered prescriber for a medication to be given to a named patient. This will include the dose, route, and frequency of the medication and could be written in the patient's notes.

Patient Group Directions

Patient group directions are legal frameworks, which allow healthcare professionals to supply/administer medication to a predefined group, e.g. 1 g paracetamol for pyretic patients. The PGDs should be produced by a senior doctor/dentist and a pharmacist and those using it must be authorised to administer medication. They must also be named and authorised to practise under it; this will include training and assessment of competency.

NB: As with all medications you need to have the necessary professional skills and knowledge of the medication and be competent in the use of electronic systems as required.

Key Legislation in Medication Administration

- Medicines Act 1968 (as amended).
- The Misuse of Drugs Act 1971.
- The Misuse of Drugs Regulations 1973.
- POM Order 1983 (as amended).
- Patient Group Directions (2000).
- Human Medicines Regulations (2012).

Red Flags

- Similarly named patients.
- Similarly named medications.
- Inappropriate route for patient.
- Adverse reactions.

References

Elliot, M. and Liu, Y. (2010). The nine rights of medication administration: an overview. *British Journal of Nursing* 2010 (19): 5300–5305.

Medicines and Healthcare products Regulatory Agency (2012). *Medicines and Medical Devices Regulation: What You Need to Know*. London: MHRA.

Nursing and Midwifery Council (2018). *Future Nurses: Standards of Proficiency for Registered Nurses*. London: NMC.

15 Injection technique

Figure 15.1 Anatomy and physiology of the skin.

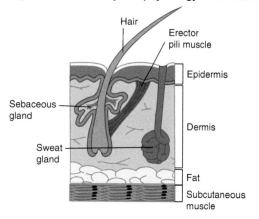

Figure 15.2 Safety needles.

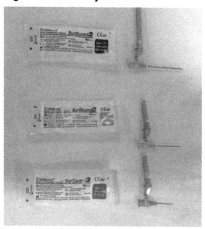

Figure 15.3 Subcutaneous injection sites.

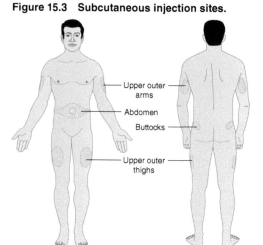

Figure 15.4 Subcutaneous injection.

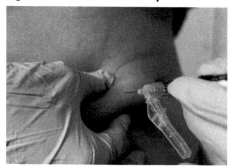

Figure 15.5 Z-track technique.

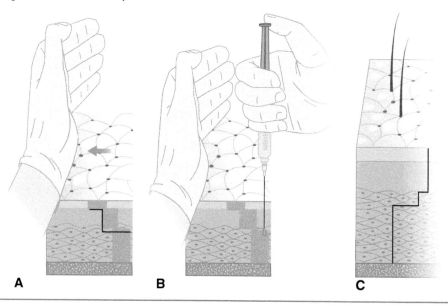

A   B   C

Clinical Nursing Skills at a Glance, First Edition. Edited by Sarah Curr and Carol Fordham-Clarke.
© 2022 John Wiley & Sons Ltd. Published 2022 by John Wiley & Sons Ltd.
Companion website: www.wiley.com/go/clinicalnursingskills

Background

- The skin has four main layers: the epidermis, the dermis, subcutaneous layer, and muscle (Figure 15.1).
- The main structures of the skin are found in the dermis where there are sweat glands, hair follicles, and a dense network of nerve endings.
- There are fewer nerve endings in the subcutaneous and muscle layers, thus making it more important to administer an injection into the correct layer of skin.
- Subcutaneous injections are administered into the subcutaneous layer.
- Intramuscular injections are administered into the muscle layer.
- Good blood flow to all layers of the skin means that medicines are absorbed quickly.

Professional Approach

- Informed consent must be obtained from patients before administering an injection. Where a patient is unable to provide this or lacks capacity, a best-interest decision should be made.
- Some patients may feel uncomfortable with exposing body parts for an injection. Privacy and dignity should be maintained throughout.
- Patients may feel anxious about needles and receiving an injection, so effective communication is essential to reduce this anxiety.

Influencing Factors

Patients could be scared, in pain, or confused when a medication is given, and needle phobias should be considered. Ultimately you need to consider why you are giving the medication via this route and if this is the most appropriate one. Medication is usually given via intramuscular or subcutaneous routes if a quicker effect is needed or if drug absorption through the stomach may be impaired.

Equipment

- Injectate in syringe of suitable size. The needle should be changed once the injectate is drawn up to avoid tracking of the injectate through the skin layers. Ideally the injectate should be drawn up with a blunt, drawing-up needle, before changing to the needle for injection.
- Needle size depends on route and patient size (Figure 15.2):
  - For a subcutaneous injection, a 23 or 25G needle should suffice.
  - Pre-filled subcutaneous syringes are usually 29G.
  - For an intramuscular injection, a 21G needle is usual.
- Sharps container.
- Clean tray to carry equipment.
- Gloves may be required (refer to local policy).

Procedure

- Prepare your equipment.
- Obtain informed consent.

- Wash hands or decontaminate with alcohol rub.
- Consider applying gloves (refer to local policy).
- Identify a suitable site and ensure that the drug is licensed for administration into that site.
- If giving an injection into visible soiled skin, cleanse the skin using soap and water then allow to dry.
- If administering a subcutaneous injection, pinch up at the chosen site to move the subcutaneous layer away from the muscle (Figures 15.3 and 15.4).
- If administering an intramuscular injection, use a Z-track technique (Figure 15.5) (Yilmaz et al. 2016) to avoid injectate seeping back out along the needle track.
- Administer injections using a 90° angle for both subcutaneous and intramuscular injections unless clinical judgement indicates otherwise.
- Depress plunger of syringe slowly until injectate has been delivered in full.
- Remove needle 10 seconds after injectate has been delivered and release skin.
- Employ the safety mechanism and dispose of the needle in the sharps container immediately.
- Do not massage the skin unless indicated by the drug licensure.

Procedure – Which Intramuscular Site

Table 15.1

Red Flags

- ▶ If the site appears oedematous or bruised or skin is broken, use a different site.
- ▶ If blood appears in the syringe, a blood vessel could have been punctured; do not inject, withdraw the needle immediately, and apply pressure.
- ▶ If the patient is agitated or uncooperative, assess the situation carefully due to risk of sharps injury.
- ▶ If the patient complains of feeling itchy or nauseated or they appear unwell, suspect allergic reaction and treat immediately.

References

Greenway, K. (2014). Rituals in nursing: intramuscular injection. *Journal of Clinical Nursing* 23 (24): 3583–3588.

Kaya, N., Salmaslioglu, A., Terzi, B. et al. (2015). The reliability of site determination methods on ventrogluteal are injection: a cross sectional study. *International Journal of Nursing Studies* 52 (1): 355–360.

Larkin, T.A., Ashcroft, E., Hickey, B.A., and Elgellaie, A. (2018). Influence of gender, BMI and body shape on theoretical injection outcome at the ventrogluteal and dorsogluteal sites. *Journal of Clinical Nursing* 27 (1): e242–e250.

Yilmaz, D., Khorshid, L., and Dedeoguy, Y. (2016). The effect of the Z-track technique on pain and drug leakage in intramuscular injection. *Clinical Nurse Specialist.* 30 (6): E7–E12.

Table 15.1 Intramuscular injection sites.

Dorsogluteal	No longer recommended as it is close to sciatic nerve and gluteal artery. Rise in obesity (body mass index > 24.9 kg/m²) means it is less likely injectate will reach muscle even with 21G needle (Greenway 2014)	
Ventrogluteal	Safest site, as there is less subcutaneous fat and it is away from other structures Landmark using the geometric rather than the V (Kaya et al. 2015; Larkin et al. 2018): • Draw an imaginary line from the greater trochanter to the iliac crest • Then draw the line to the anterosuperior iliac spine • Then draw line from the anterosuperior iliac spine to the greater trochanter (this produces a triangle) • Then draw lines from each corner of the triangle • Where these three lines meet is the site of injection	
Deltoid	Easily accessible	
Vastus lateralis	Good option for those with mobility problems. Can accommodate larger volumes Landmark to avoid femoral artery	

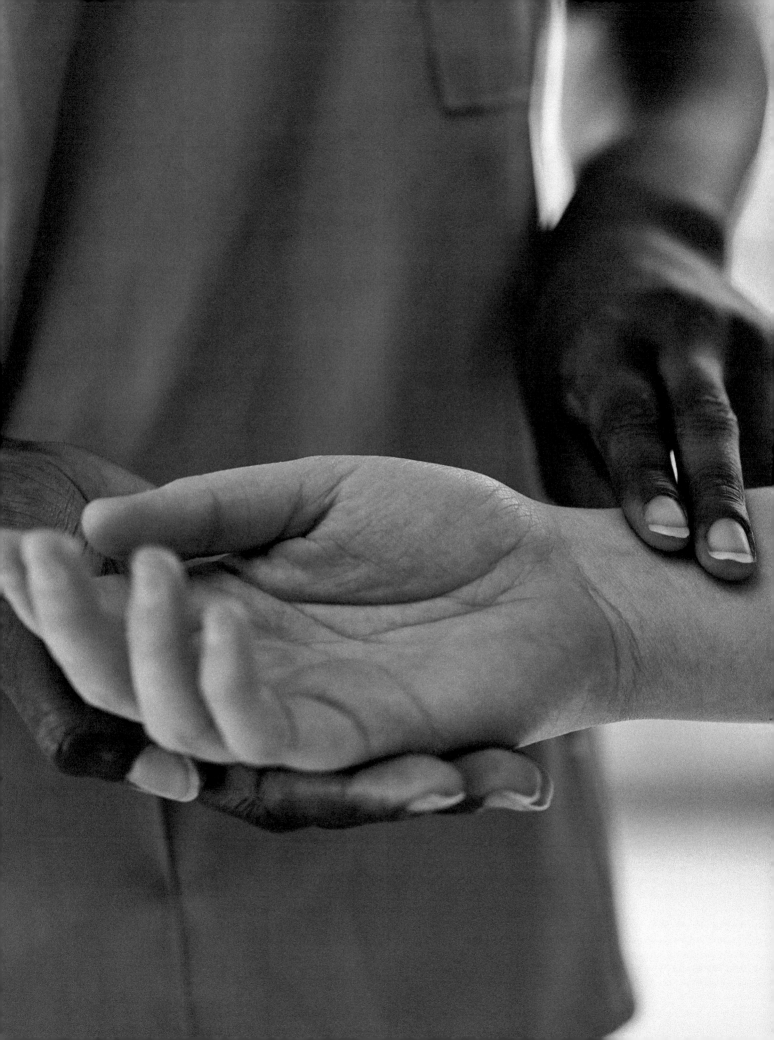

National early warning score (NEWS) track and trigger system

Figure 16.1 National Early Warning Score (NEWS 2) chart. Source: National Early Warning Score (NEWS) 2 (2017)/Royal College of Physicians.

NEWS key													
0 1 2 3	**FULL NAME**												

	DATE TIME								DATE TIME

A+B Respirations Breaths/min

				score
≥25			3	≥25
21–24			2	21–24
18–20				18–20
15–17				15–17
12–14				12–14
9–11			1	9–11
≤8			3	≤8

A+B SpO₂ Scale 1 Oxygen saturation (%)

≥96				≥96
94–95			1	94–95
92–93			2	92–93
≤91			3	≤91

SpO₂ Scale 2† Oxygen saturation (%) Use Scale 2 if target range is 88–92%, eg in hypercapnic respiratory failure. †ONLY use Scale 2 under the direction of a qualified clinician

≥97 on O₂			3	≥97 on O₂
95–96 on O₂			2	95–96 on O₂
93–94 on O₂			1	93–94 on O₂
≥93 on air				≥93 on air
88–92				88–92
86–87			1	86–87
84–85			2	84–85
≤83%			3	≤83%

Air or oxygen?

A=Air				A=Air
O₂ L/min			2	O₂ L/min
Device				Device

C Blood pressure mmHg Score uses systolic BP only

≥220			3	≥220
201–219				201–219
181–200				181–200
161–180				161–180
141–160				141–160
121–140				121–140
111–120				111–120
101–110			1	101–110
91–100			2	91–100
81–90				81–90
71–80				71–80
61–70			3	61–70
51–60				51–60
≤50				≤50

C Pulse Beats/min

≥131			3	≥131
121–130			2	121–130
111–120				111–120
101–110			1	101–110
91–100				91–100
81–90				81–90
71–80				71–80
61–70				61–70
51–60				51–60
41–50			1	41–50
31–40			3	31–40
≤30				≤30

D Consciousness Score for NEW onset of confusion (no score if chronic)

Alert				Alert
Confusion				Confusion
V			3	V
P				P
U				U

E Temperature °C

≥39.1°			2	≥39.1°
38.1–39.0°			1	38.1–39.0°
37.1–38.0°				37.1–38.0°
36.1–37.0°				36.1–37.0°
35.1–36.0°			1	35.1–36.0°
≤35.0°			3	≤35.0°

NEWS TOTAL					TOTAL
Monitoring frequency					Monitoring
Escalation of care Y/N					Escalation
Initials					Initials

National Early Warning Score 2 (NEWS2) © Royal College of Physicians 2017

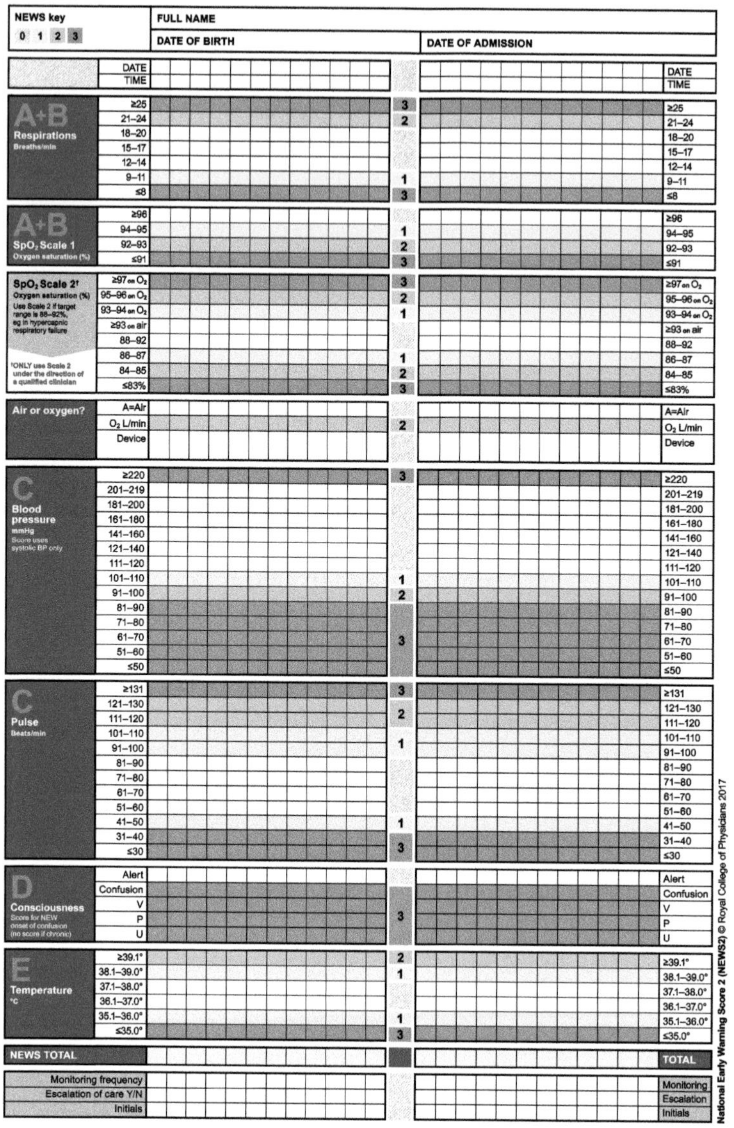

Figure 16.2 Oxygen usage using the Royal College of Physicians abbreviations.

Abbreviation	Full Meaning
A	Air Breathing
N	Nasal Cannula
SM	Simple face mask
V24	Venturi Mask and percentage, in this case 24%
NIV	Non-invasive ventilation
RM	Reservoir Mask
TM	Tracheostomy mask
CP	Continuous positive airway pressure (CPAP) mask
H28	Humidified Oxygen and percentage, in this case 28%
OTH	Other, please specific

Clinical Nursing Skills at a Glance, First Edition. Edited by Sarah Curr and Carol Fordham-Clarke.
© 2022 John Wiley & Sons Ltd. Published 2022 by John Wiley & Sons Ltd.
Companion website: www.wiley.com/go/clinicalnursingskills

Figure 16.3   National Early Warning Score (NEWS) scoring. *Source*: **National Early Warning Score (NEWS) 2 (2017)/Royal College of Physicians.**

NEW score	Frequency of monitoring	Clinical response
0	Minimum 12 hourl	• Continue routine NEWS monitoring
Total 1–4	Minimum 4–6 hourly	• Inform registered nurse, who must assess the patient • Registered nurse decides whether increased frequency of monitoring and/or escalation of care are required
3 in single parameter	Minimum 1 hourly	• Registered nurse to inform medical team caring for the patient, who will review and decide whether escalation of care is necessary
Total 5 or more Urgent response threshold	Minimum 1 hourly	• Registered nurse to immediately inform the medical team caring for the patient • Registered nurse to request urgent assessment by a clinician or team with core competencies in the care of acutely ill patients • Provide clinical care in an environment with monitoring facilities
Total 7 or more Emergency response threshold	Continuous monitoring of vital signs	• Registered nurse to immediately inform the medical team caring for the patient – this should be at least at specialist registrar level • Emergency assessment by a team with critical care competencies, including practitioner(s) with advanced airway management skills • Consider transfer of care to a level 2 or 3 clinical care facility, ie higher-dependency unit or ICU • Clinical care in an environment with monitoring facilities

Figure 16.4   Escalation to the designated clinical personnel. *Source*: **National Early Warning Score (NEWS) 2 (2017)/Royal College of Physicians.**

NEW score	Clinical risk	Response
Aggregate score 0–4	Low	Ward-based response
Red score Score of 3 in any individual parameter	Low–medium	Urgent ward-based response*
Aggregate score 5–6	Medium	Key threshold for urgent response*
Aggregate score 7 or more	High	Urgent or emergency response**

* Response by a clinician or team with competence in the assessment and treatment of acutely ill patients and in recognising when the escalation of care to a critical care team is appropriate.

**The response team must also include staff with critical care skills, including airway management.

Background

In order to recognise the acutely ill adult, various track and trigger systems have been used in the clinical setting. In 2012 the Royal College of Physicians (RCP) in the United Kingdom implemented a nationwide early warning scoring system, the National Early Warning Score (NEWS) (RCP 2012) to ensure consistency in track and trigger systems across healthcare providers. The NEWS, now NEWS 2 (Figure 16.1), is used widely within secondary care but has also been adopted in the out-of-hospital setting and internationally (RCP 2017). This system provides standardisation of clinical monitoring, a clear guide for clinical response, highlights when escalation to higher dependency and care intensity settings is required, while also providing guidance on the frequency of monitoring of vital signs.

Professional Approach

- In order to use the NEWS, the healthcare professional must be trained and deemed competent. As such it is recommended that prior to performance of this skill the RCP e-learning NEWS package is completed, followed by a period of supervised practice to ensure competency.
- Before undertaking the A–E NEWS assessment, the patient must be informed of all elements of the assessment and provided with an adequate rationale as to why it is performed in order that informed consent can be given.
- To ensure safe practice, all individuals who undertake these measurements and use the NEWS must be familiar with normal and abnormal parameters and recognise individual factors that may affect scoring, e.g. SpO_2 scale 2 for those with hypercapnic respiratory failure.
- For each assessment, the healthcare professional must perform all vital signs and ensure full completion of the chart before calculating the NEWS and potentially escalating care.
- During measurement, documentation, and escalation the patient must be informed of all decisions made and potential next steps.

NB: Remember that it is essential to act within your competency when measuring and observing the patient's vital signs. Although interventions are encouraged, only those that sit within your professional scope of practice should be undertaken. The exception to this are actions that are undertaken in an emergency (National Institute of Health and Care Excellence 2007).

Influencing Factors

- Triggering on the NEWS occurs due to vital signs that sit outside of the normal range. The RCP recognises that this is usually as a result of physiological changes in the acutely unwell adult (RCP 2017). As such it is important to remember that this assessment is used for the scoring of the acutely unwell adult and is not intended to replace the holistic assessment undertaken on admission to a care setting.
- Do remember that in some instances there may be a concern that is not reflected by a trigger on the scoring system. In such circumstances individual clinical judgement should be used (RCP 2012).

- Whilst the NEWS is nationwide and used internationally, escalation will be specific to the organisation in which you work and thus familiarisation of organisation guidance and policy, to ensure correct escalation, will also be required.

Equipment

- All equipment required for the separate vital signs to be measured.
- NEWS chart, either electronic or paper copy.

Procedure

- Prepare your equipment.
- Gain informed consent.
- Wash hands or decontaminate with alcohol hand rub.
- Follow the ABCDE approach (Resuscitation Council UK 2021) outlined on the chart.
- Note all vital signs clearly and accurately.
- Note oxygen usage using the RCP (2017) recognised abbreviations (Figure 16.2).
- Once all measurements are completed and documented, calculate NEWS.
- Note if patient score represents a low, medium or high risk of clinical deterioration (Figure 16.3).
- Escalate to the designated clinical personnel (Figure 16.4).

NB: Remember that an A–E assessment requires both measurement and monitoring of vital signs but also timely interventions to prevent further deterioration. These interventions should be commenced after each measurement and reassessed for effect prior to escalation of care.

Red Flags

▸ Be aware that NEWS is not reliable when assessing those with spinal injuries.

▸ Remember that NEWS is only suitable for use on adults over 16 years of age.

▸ Do not use NEWS on pregnant women as their vital signs fall outside of the normal parameters.

▸ There are specific NEWS charts available for paediatrics and obstetrics.

References

Monsieurs, K.G., Nolan, J.P., Bossaert, L.L. et al. (2015). European Resuscitation Council guidelines for resuscitation 2015 section 1. Executive summary. *Resuscitation* 95: 1–80.

National Institute of Health and Care Excellence (2007). *CG50 Acutely Ill Adults in Hospital: Recognising and Responding to Deterioration.* London: National Institute of Health and Care Excellence.

Resuscitation Council UK 2021 *Resuscitation Guidelines: The ABCDE Approach.* https://www.resus.org.uk/library/abcde-approach.

Royal College of Physicians (2017). *National Early Warning Score (NEWS) 2: Standardising the Assessment of Acute Illness Severity in the NHS. Report of a Working Party.* London: Royal College of Physicians.

Royal College of Physicians (RCP) (2012). *National Early Warning Score (NEWS) 2: Standardising the Assessment of Acute Illness Severity in the NHS. Report of a Working Party.* London: Royal College of Physicians.

Neurological skills

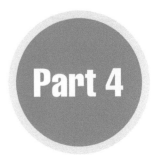

Part 4

Chapters

17 Assessing level of consciousness

Figure 17.1 ACVPU recording.

	Alert		
Consciousness	Confusion		
Score for NEW	V		
onset of confusion	P		
(no score if chronic)	U		

Table 17.1 The ACVPU assessment tool.

Assessment	Response
Alert	The person is fully awake, eyes open, and able to move and respond appropriately
Confusion	Coherent but inappropriate, unoriented response
Voice	Any kind of response to the sound of voice, but without being fully awake
Pain	Any kind of response to a painful stimulus
Unresponsive	No eye, verbal, or motor responses to pain stimuli

Table 17.2 Structured assessment of Glasgow Coma Scale (GCS).

Check	For factors that can interfere with ability to communicate
Observe	Eye opening, verbal and motor response
Stimulate	Sound; a spoken or shouted request Pressure; on fingertip, trapezius or supraorbital notch
Rate	Record best response

Table 17.3 The Glasgow Coma Scale (GCS) assessment tool.

Assessment	Rating	Score	Response
Eye response	Spontaneous	E4	Open before stimulus
	To sound	E3	Open after spoken or shouted request
	To pressure	E2	Open in response to application of pressure to the lateral aspect of the finger or fingernail (Figure 17.2)
	None	E1	No opening at any time and no interfering factors. Ensure that pressure has increased over the 10-second period and is an adequate pressure before recording as E1
	Non-testable	NT	Closed due to local factors, e.g. swelling
Verbal response	Orientated	V5	Orientated to name, place, and date
	Confused	V4	Not orientated, communicates coherently
	Words	V3	Intelligible single words
	Sounds	V2	Moans and groans
	None	V1	No audible response and interfering factor
	Non-testable	NT	Factors influencing communication
Motor response	Obeys commands	M6	Obeys two-part request
	Localising	M5	Brings hands above clavicle to central stimulus
	Normal flexion	M4	Bends arm at elbow rapidly but does not appear abnormal
	Abnormal flexion	M3	Bends arm at elbow abnormally
	Extension	M2	Extends arm at elbow
	None	M1	No movement in limbs and no interfering factors
	Non-testable	NT	Due to factors influencing movement, e.g. paralysis

NB: If there are different responses from the right and left sides of the body, record the best response.

Source: Adapted from Teasdale et al. (2014).

Figure 17.2 Applying pressure: fingernail.

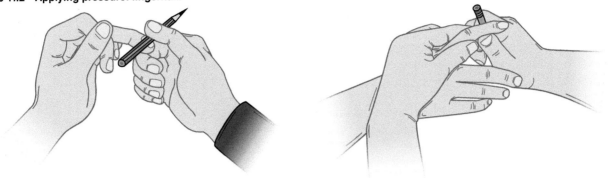

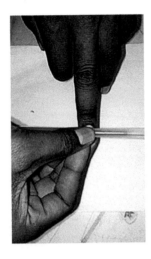

Figure 17.3 Applying pressure: trapezium pinch.

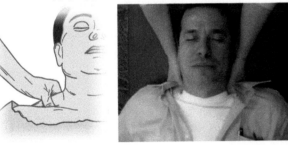

Figure 17.4 Applying pressure: supraorbital pressure.

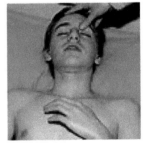

Figure 17.5 Abnormal motor responses.

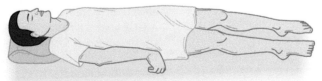

A Extension posturing (decerebrate rigidity)

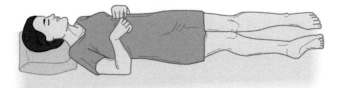

B Abnormal flexion (decorticate rigidity)

Background

- Level of consciousness measures a person's responsiveness to environmental stimuli and is a measure of overall neurological function.
- Consciousness is dependent upon arousal and awareness.
- Arousal is determined by a functioning reticular activating system (RAS) within the brain stem.
- Awareness is determined by the cerebral cortex processing information.
- Many factors can alter the level of consciousness, such as alcohol consumption, drugs, raised intracranial pressure, decreased oxygen or blood flow to the brain, hypoglycaemia, and electrolyte imbalance – in particular, sodium.
- Two tools are commonly used in clinical practice to assess consciousness: ACVPU (alert, confusion, verbal, pain, unresponsive) and Glasgow Coma Scale (GCS) (Kelly et al. 2005).

Influencing Factors

- Intoxication.
- Some drugs and medications.
- Existing disability.
- Post-ictal (post-seizure) drowsiness.
- Sleep disorders and consequent drowsiness.
- Eyes closed by swelling.
- Presence of endotracheal tube or tracheostomy.
- Communication problems.

Professional Approach

- Communicate clearly with the patient, and obtain informed consent when possible.
- Use the most appropriate assessment tool for the patient, remembering that a full neurological assessment includes:
  - GCS.
  - Limb movement and strength.
  - Pupil size and reaction to light (Chapter 18).
  - Full vital signs (Chapter 16).
- Be aware of the previous recording and baseline assessment.
- Accurate record keeping is essential, including areas that are unable to be assessed for a patient.
- Escalate changes in level of consciousness immediately to allow for early intervention.
- People sometimes require neurological observation at specific time intervals. It is important to be accurate with the required timings and follow local Trust guidance.

Equipment – The ACVPU Tool

This is commonly used by following the section on the National Early Warning Score 2 (NEWS 2) chart (Royal College of Physicians 2017) (Figure 17.1).

Procedure – The ACVPU Tool

- The ACVPU is a tool for rapid assessment and is not suitable for a detailed assessment of consciousness.
- Responses can be alert (eyes opening), verbal (response to voice command) or motor (response to stimulus).
- "New confusion" is an additional response that has been added, which changed the abbreviation AVPU to ACVPU (Royal College of Physicians 2017) (Table 17.1).

- New confusion in an otherwise alert patient is a warning sign of serious underlying illness.

Equipment – Glasgow Coma Scale

Refer to local neurological guidance.

Procedure – Glasgow Coma Scale

- This a structured assessment that must follow specific steps (Tables 17.2 and 17.3; Teasdale et al. 2014).
- Detailed scores for each response (as outlined in Table 17.3) are required and as they provide detailed information on consciousness they are more useful for diagnostic purposes.
- An overall total score of between 3 and 15 indicates severity (Table 17.3).

Procedure

- Where possible, explain the assessment to the patient to obtain informed consent.
- Initially assess for spontaneous behaviour.
- If the patient is not alert or awake, talk to them, asking them to open their eyes – this is to assess the arousal mechanisms in the brain stem (RAS).
- Table 17.3 details the full approach to follow for "eyes opening".
- Then move to check for verbal response and thus level of consciousness.
- Check orientation by asking their name, where they are and the month (Table 17.3).
- Finally assess motor response by asking the patient to grasp and release your hand or open their mouth and stick their tongue out.
- If the patient does not obey commands and there is no response, apply increasing pressure to the trapezius muscle (Figure 17.3) for up to 10 seconds.
- If this stimulus does not elicit a localising response, apply pressure to the supraorbital notch (Figure 17.4) to distinguish between the motor responses: flexion, abnormal flexion, and extension (Figure 17.5).
- Remember to record eyes, verbal, and motor separately, as well as the total score (Table 17.3).
- Escalate as appropriate.

NB: When checking conscious level, ascertain that the patient can understand English (or the language you are speaking in).

Red Flags

- Avoid applying supraorbital pressure (as a central painful stimulus) if there are any injuries to the face.
- A GCS score ≤ 8 requires intubation to maintain the airway.
- Unconsciousness following a head injury is an emergency.
- Duration of altered consciousness is associated with increased morbidity and mortality.

References

Kelly, C.A., Upex, A., and Bateman, D.N. (2005). Comparison of consciousness level assessment in the poisoned patient using the alert/verbal/painful/unresponsive scale and the Glasgow Coma Scale. *Annuals of Emergency Medicine* 44 (2): 108–113.

Royal College of Physicians (2017). *National Early Warning Score (NEWS) 2: Standardising the Assessment of Acute Illness Severity in the NHS*. London: Royal College of Physicians.

Teasdale, G., Allen, D., Brennan, P. et al. (2014). The Glasgow Coma Scale: an update after 40 years. *Nursing Times* (110): 12–16.

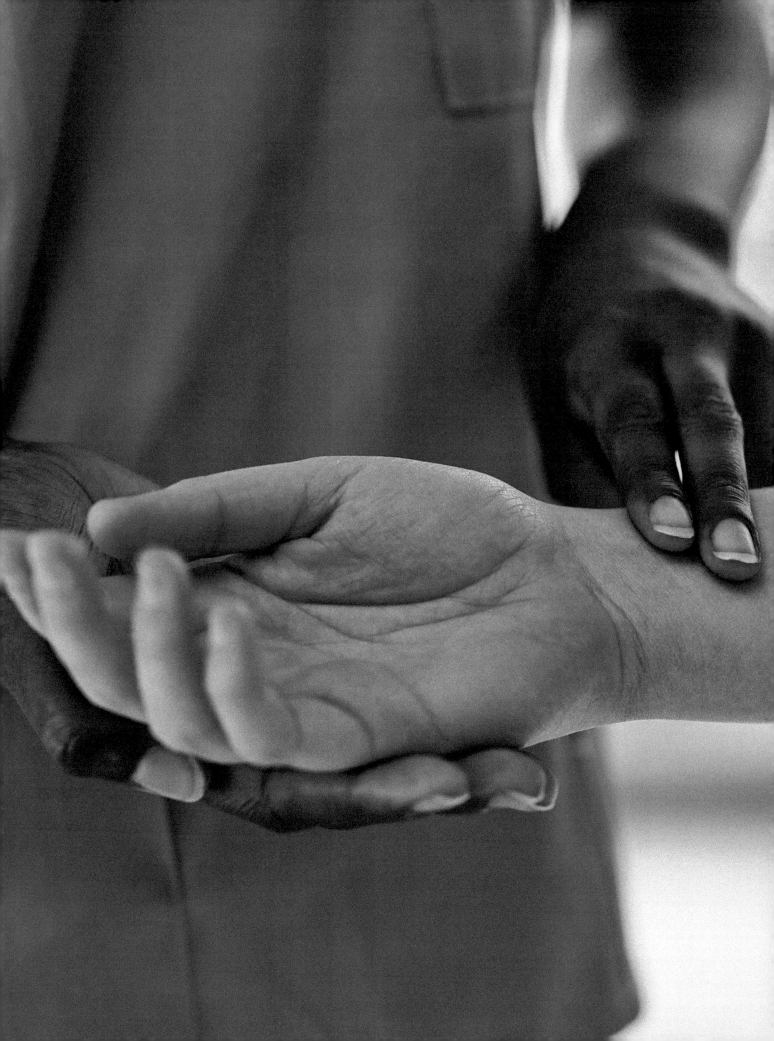

18 Assessing pupil reaction and limb strength

Figure 18.1 Pupil gauge.

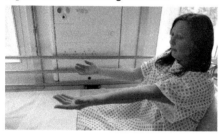

No SIM	3:37 PM	
1mm •	6mm ●	
2mm ●	7mm ●	
3mm ●	8mm ●	
4mm ●	9mm ●	
5mm ●	10mm ●	

Figure 18.2 Assessing arm drift.

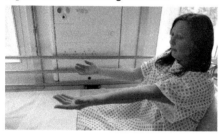

Table 18.1 Pupil reactivity score.

Pupil unreactive to light	Score
Both pupils	2
One pupil	1
Neither pupil	0

Source: Adapted from Brennan et al. (2018).

Figure 18.3 Assessing arm strength.

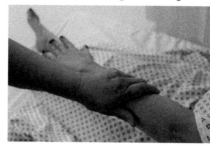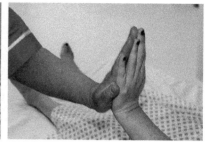

Figure 18.4 Assessing leg strength.

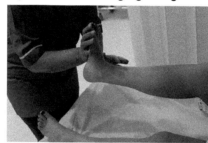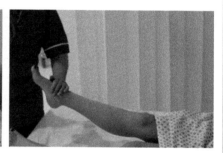

Table 18.2 Assessing limb strength.

Strength	Description
5. Normal power	Can overcome examiners strength
4. Active movement against gravity and resistance	Slight weakness – can move against resistance Drift may be noted
3. Active movement against gravity	Moderate weakness – can move against gravity but not resistance
2. Active movement with gravity eliminated	Severe Weakness – cannot move against gravity or resistance
1. Flicker or trace of contraction	Severe weakness – may be a flicker of movement
0. No contraction	Paralysis

Source: Adapted from the Medical Research Council (1976).

Clinical Nursing Skills at a Glance, First Edition. Edited by Sarah Curr and Carol Fordham-Clarke.
© 2022 John Wiley & Sons Ltd. Published 2022 by John Wiley & Sons Ltd.
Companion website: www.wiley.com/go/clinicalnursingskills

Background

- Assessing pupil size and limb strength is typically part of completing full neurological observations, along with the assessment of consciousness.
- Assessment of pupil size and reaction looks at the function of the oculomotor nerve and therefore gives an indication of intracranial pressure.
- Pupils should constrict in the presence of bright light.
- Assessing limb strength can provide information about both the brain and spinal cord.

Influencing Factors

- Medications altering pupil size.
- Existing eye injury or condition.
- Eyes closed by swelling.
- Existing injury or disability affecting any limb.
- Difficulty understanding or acting on instructions for any reason.

Professional Approach

- Accurate record keeping is essential.
- Rapid reporting of changes can prevent deterioration.
- People sometimes require neurological observation at specific time intervals. It is important to be accurate with the required timings.
- People with brain injuries or migraine may be light-sensitive; consider whether pain relief will be needed prior to assessment.

Procedure – Assessing Pupil Reactivity Score

- First, assess and compare the size and shape of the pupils – measure the size in mm, using a pupil gauge (Figure 18.1).
- Using a pen torch, sweep the light from the outer edge towards the nose.
- Observe the pupil of that eye for a reaction.
- Observe the pupil of the other eye for a reaction – the reactions should be identical.
- Repeat the procedure in the other eye.
- Document the size of each pupil initially at rest and whether there was a reaction to light – if so, was it brisk or sluggish?
- This needs to be documented according to local policy; common systems are + and – or R and N for reaction or no reaction, respectively, and S for sluggish.
- A hippus reaction may be seen, where the size of the pupil oscillates in response to light. This is seen in some neurological conditions and is often recorded as H.

Subtracting the pupil reactivity score from the Glasgow Coma Scale can be used as an indicator of severity of traumatic brain injury (Table 18.1).

Procedure – Assessing Limb Strength

- This guide is for the care of conscious patients; limb assessment is different in unconscious patients.

- A simple test for equality of arm strength is to ask the patient to hold their arms out in front of them at 90° with palms up and to close their eyes. If either arm drifts downwards within two minutes, weakness is present (Figure 18.2).
- The following, more detailed assessment can be used to assess range of movement and strength. Where resistance is needed, use your own hand and only enough pressure to assess that the person can push against you.
- To assess the arms:
  - Ask the patient to flex at the elbow and straighten the arm with and without resistance.
  - Ask the patient to raise the shoulders without and against resistance, then lower them.
  - Ask the patient to push against your hand (Figure 18.3).
  - Check for differences between each side.
- To assess the legs (Figure 18.4):
  - Ask the patient to lift their straightened leg against gravity.
  - Ask the patient to lift their leg whilst downward pressure is applied to the leg.
  - Ask the patient to flex the foot towards the shin (dorsiflexion).
  - Ask the patient to extend the foot, pointing the toes (plantar flexion).
  - Check for differences between each side.
- Record the results. Many neurological observation charts contain boxes to record power in arms and legs as normal, mild weakness, severe weakness or no movement, and Table 18.2 provides further guidance on this. A more detailed description of deficits should also be recorded in the patient's notes.

Red Flags

- Differentiate between limbs when recording on the chart if different responses are obtained from right and left sides.
- Decreased pupil reaction coupled with increasing pupillary size, sometimes with unequal pupils, can be a sign of rising intracranial pressure.
- Changes in pupil size and reaction and/or limb power must be escalated to the appropriate personnel immediately.
- Unequal limb power can indicate damage to one hemisphere of the brain and can be sudden in stroke.

References

Brennan, P.M., Murray, G.D., and Teasdale, G.M. (2018). Simplifying the use of prognostic information in traumatic brain injury. Part 1: the GSC-pupils score: an extended index of clinical severity. *Journal of Neurosurgery* 128 (6): 1612–1620.

Medical Research Council (1976) *Memorandum No. 45. Aids to the Examination of the Peripheral Nervous System.* https://mrc.ukri.org/documents/pdf/aids-to-the-examination-of-the-peripheral-nervous-system-mrc-memorandum-no-45-superseding-war-memorandum-no-7

19 Assessing cognition

Figure 19.1 Mini-Mental State Examination – sample questions.

MMSE SAMPLE ITEMS

ORIENTATION TO TIME

"What is the date?"

REGISTRATION

"Listen carefully. I am going to say three words. You say them back after I stop.

Ready? Here they are…

APPLE (pause), PENNY(pause), TABLE(pause). Now repeat those words back to me."
[Repeat up to 5 times, but score only the first trial.]

NAMING

"What is this?" [Point to a pencil or pen.]

READING

"Please read this and do what it says." [Show examinee the words on the stimulus form.]

CLOSE YOUR EYES

Source: Reproduced by special permission of the Publisher, Psychological Assessment Resources, Inc., 16204 North Florida Avenue, Lutz, Florida 33549, from the Mini Mental State Examination, by Marshal Folstein and Susan Folstein, Copyright 1975, 1998, 2001 by MiniMental LLC, Inc. Published 2001 by Psychological Assessment Resources, Inc. Further reproduction is prohibited without permission of PAR, Inc. The MMSE can be purchased from PAR, Inc. by calling (813) 968-3003.

Figure 19.2 Confusion Assessment Method (CAM) – short form. *Source:* © 2003, Hospital Elder Life Program, LLC.

CONFUSION ASSESSMENT METHOD (CAM) ALGORITHM

(1) acute onset and fluctuating course

-and-

(2) inattention

-and either-

(3) disorganized thinking

-or-

(4) altered level of consciousness

[Score based on cognitive testing. See details at:
www.hospitalelderlifeprogram.org]

Copyright © 2003 Hospital Elder Life Program, LLC. All rights reserved.

Figure 19.3 Mini-Cog. *Source:* Mini-Cog© Instructions for Administration & Scoring/Mini-Cog © S. Borson.

Mini-Cog™ Instructions for Administration & Scoring
ID _____ Date: _____

Step 1: Three Word Registration

Look directly at person and say, "Please listen carefully. I am going to say three words that I want you to repeat back to me now and try to remember. The words are [select a list of words from the versions below]. Please say them for me now." If the person is unable to repeat the words after three attempts, move on to Step 2 (clock drawing).

The following and other word lists have been used in one or more clinical studies.[1] For repeated administrations, use of an alternative word list is recommended.

Version 1	Version 2	Version 3	Version 4	Version 5	Version 6
Banana	Leader	Village	River	Captain	Daughter
Sunrise	Season	Kitchen	Nation	Garden	Heaven
Chair	Table	Baby	Finger	Picture	Mountain

Step 2: Clock Drawing

Say: "Next, I want you to draw a clock for me. First, put in all of the numbers where they go." When that is completed, say: "Now, set the hands to 10 past 11."

Use preprinted circle (see next page) for this exercise. Repeat instructions as needed as this is not a memory test. Move to Step 3 if the clock is not complete within three minutes.

Step 3: Three Word Recall

Ask the person to recall the three words you stated in Step 1. Say: "What were the three words I asked you to remember?" Record the word list version number and the person's answers below.

Word List Version: _____ Person's Answers: _____

Scoring

Word Recall:	_____ (0-3 points)	1 point for each word spontaneously recalled without cueing.
Clock Draw:	_____ (0 or 2 points)	Normal clock = 2 points. A normal clock has all numbers placed in the correct sequence and approximately correct position (e.g. 12, 3, 6 and 9 are in anchor positions) with no missing or duplicate numbers. Hands are pointing to the 11 and 2 (10:10). Hand length is not scored. Inability or refusal to draw a clock (abnormal) = 0 points.
Total Score:	_____ (0-5 points)	Total score = Word Recall score + Clock Draw score. A cut point of <3 on the Mini-Cog™ has been validated for dementia screening, but many individuals with clinically meaningful cognitive impairment will score higher. When greater sensitivity is desired, a cut point of <4 is recommended as it may indicate a need for further evaluation of cognitive status.

Mini-Cog™ © S. Borson. All rights reserved. Reprinted with permission of the author solely for clinical and educational purposes. May not be modified or used for commercial, marketing, or research purposes without permission of the author (soob@uw.edu).

Clinical Nursing Skills at a Glance, First Edition. Edited by Sarah Curr and Carol Fordham-Clarke.
© 2022 John Wiley & Sons Ltd. Published 2022 by John Wiley & Sons Ltd.
Companion website: www.wiley.com/go/clinicalnursingskills

Background

- Assessing cognition encompasses assessments of memory, orientation, language, mood, and executive functioning.
- Delirium and dementia share many of the same symptoms. Delirium comes on quickly generally due to an acute health problem and resolves with management, whereas dementia typically appears over a longer period of time and cannot be reversed.
- In dementia changes can be linked to specific areas of the brain: e.g. problems with visual processing or memory can indicate damage to the occipital lobe, and problems with mood can indicate frontal lobe problems.
- A full cognitive assessment can take an hour, so the Mini-Mental State Examination (MMSE) (Folstein et al. 1975) is often used.
- The short Confusion Assessment Method (CAM) (Inouye et al. 1990) can also be used when dementia is suspected.
- It is often impractical to assess all areas of cognition, and thus a knowledge of the patient's history is important.

Influencing Factors

- Existing disabilities or long-term illnesses.
- Recent head injury.
- Problems with communication. This includes hearing aids, which can exacerbate signs of dementia if not working effectively
- Unable or unwilling to cooperate.
- Medications that cause drowsiness or affect cognition.
- Disorientation to place and time exacerbated by hospitalisation.

With delirium there are specific risk factors that indicate the need for further testing (NICE 2019):

- Age 65+.
- Existing cognitive impairment and/or dementia.
- Hip fracture.
- Severe illness.

Professional Approach

- Explain what you are examining and how long it will take to ensure informed consent is obtained.
- Consider taking the person to a quieter area. If not available, consider how to reduce noise and distractions.

Equipment – MMSE

- Ensure that your copy of the test consists of 11 questions and problems, which assess:
  - Orientation (Figure 19.1).
  - Registration (Figure 19.1).
  - Attention and calculation.
  - Recall (Figure 19.1).
  - Language.
- Ensure that the test used is in accordance with local Trust policy – examples of MMSE test questions can be found in Figure 19.1.

Procedure – MMSE

- Complete all 11 items.
- Calculate the score.
- The 11 items provide a score out of 30, with any score > 27 being considered normal cognition.
- Low scores correlate closely with dementia; however, a high score does not exclude this.
- In patients with low educational attainment or specific learning disabilities, certain tests may need to be adjusted or interpreted differently.

- In patients for whom English is a second or other language, serial sevens is considered more appropriate than backwards spelling.

Equipment – CAM – Short Form

- Use the recognised short CAM (Inouye et al. 1990) (in accordance with local Trust policy and level of training.
- There are four features (Figure 19.2):
  1 Acute onset and fluctuating course.
  2 Inattention.
  3 Disorganised thinking.
  4 Altered level of conscious.

Procedure – CAM – Short Form

- Ask the patient and family members, friends, and significant others if:
- there has been an acute onset.
- it fluctuates throughout the day.
- there is any inattention, i.e. difficulty focusing.
- the patient is experiencing disorganised thinking, i.e. switching from topic to topic.
- Assess level of consciousness.
- Score the four features. Diagnosis of delirium requires a positive result in 1, 2, and 3 or 4 alone.

Equipment – The Mini-Cog

Use the recognised tool (Borson et al. 2003) for screening for cognition impairment in older adults when dementia is suspected (NICE 2018)

Procedure – The Mini-Cog

- This involves three steps (Figure 19.3):
  1 Three-word registration.
  2 Clock drawing.
  3 Three-word recall.
- Ensure that all steps are followed in order and marked out of 10. A person is considered likely to have dementia if they score ≤ 3 with an abnormal clock drawing.

Red Flags

- Rapid changes can indicate neurological changes such as raised intracranial pressure.
- Delirium can be a result of critical illness, and any new onset of confusion must be assessed in line with all vital signs and escalated appropriately.

References

Borson, S., Scanlon, J.M., Chen, P., and Ganguli, M. (2003). The mini-cog as a screen for dementia: validation in a population based sample. *Journal of the American Geriatric Society SI* 10: 1451–1454.

Folstein, M.F., Folstein, S.E., and McHugh, P.R. (1975). Mini-mental state. A practical method for grading the cognitive state of patients for the clinician. *Journal of Psychiatric Research* 12 (3): 189–198.

Inouye, S.K., van Dyck, C.H., Balkins, S. et al. (1990). Clarifying confusion: the confusion assessment method. A new method for detection of delirium. *Annuals of Internal Medicine* 113 (12): 941–948.

NICE (2019). *Delirium: Prevention, Diagnosis, and Management Clinical Guideline [CG103]*. London: National Institute for Health and Care Excellence.

NICE (2018). *Dementia: Assessment, Management and Support for People Living with Dementia and their Carers. NICE Guideline [NG97]*. London: National Institute for Health and Care Excellence.

20 Pain assessment

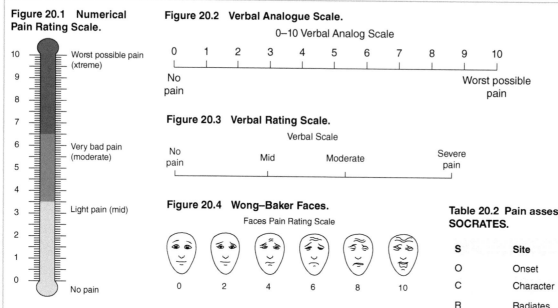

Figure 20.1 Numerical Pain Rating Scale.

- 10 — Worst possible pain (xtreme)
- 9
- 8
- 7
- 6 — Very bad pain (moderate)
- 5
- 4
- 3 — Light pain (mid)
- 2
- 1
- 0
- No pain

Figure 20.2 Verbal Analogue Scale.

0–10 Verbal Analog Scale

0 1 2 3 4 5 6 7 8 9 10

No pain   Worst possible pain

Figure 20.3 Verbal Rating Scale.

Verbal Scale

No pain   Mid   Moderate   Severe pain

Figure 20.4 Wong–Baker Faces.

Faces Pain Rating Scale

0   2   4   6   8   10

Table 20.2 Pain assessment using SOCRATES.

S	Site
O	Onset
C	Character
R	Radiates
A	Associated symptoms
T	Time/duration
E	Exacerbating/relieving factors
S	Severity

Table 20.1 Assess the characteristics of pain using PQRST.

P	Provokes	What makes the pain better/worse?
Q	Quality	What does the pain feel like?
R	Radiates	Where is the pain felt?
S	Severity	How bad is the pain?
T	Time	How long does the pain last?

Table 20.3 PAINAD assessment tool.

PAINAD score				
Items	0	1	2	Score
Breathing independent of vocalisation	Normal	Occasional laboured breathing Short period of hyperventilation	Noisy labored breathing Long period of hyperventilation Cheyne–Stokes respirations	
Negative vocalisation	None	Occasional moan or groan Low-level speech with a negative or disapproving quality	Repeated troubled calling out Loud moaning or groaning Crying	
Facial expression	Smiling or inexpressive	Sad Frightened Frown	Facial grimacing	
Body language	Relaxed	Tense Distressed pacing Fidgeting	Rigid Fists clenched Knees pulled up Pulling or pushing away Striking out	
Consolability	No need to console	Distracted or reassured by voice or touch	Unable to console, distract or reassure	
Total				

Clinical Nursing Skills at a Glance, First Edition. Edited by Sarah Curr and Carol Fordham-Clarke.
© 2022 John Wiley & Sons Ltd. Published 2022 by John Wiley & Sons Ltd.
Companion website: www.wiley.com/go/clinicalnursingskills

Background

- The experience of pain is physiologically complex involving the central and peripheral nervous systems.
- Pain is often associated with acute tissue damage, but chronic pain can result from damage to nerves (neuropathic pain) or pain-regulating structures.
- Acute pain is classified as being of ≤ 3 months duration.
- Chronic pain is pain of ≥ 3 months duration.
- Greater pain is associated with emotional distress.

Influencing Factors

- Ability to understand the pain assessment and/or respond.
- Cognitive function – impacts on response and demonstration of pain.
- Level of consciousness.
- Chronic pain.
- Scale used – for consistency, use the tool recommended by your local Trust policy for the specific group you are assessing. People with reduced cognition may need specialist assessment tools.

Professional Approach

- There are numerical and visual pain scores assessing severity of pain. Ensure that the most appropriate one for the patient is used.
- Ensure that you are competent to use the tool and explain to the patient how it is used.
- Remember that personal experiences and attitudes can vary responses, and people may under- or over-report pain for many reasons, so you may need to look for other indicators, i.e. facial expressions, sweating.
- Remember that pain should be treated according to the patient's own assessment wherever possible, as this cannot be objectively, externally, measured as "Pain is what the patient says it is" (McCaffery 1968, p. 95).

Equipment – All Scoring Systems

- As pain is a subjective assessment, using self-assessment scales where possible is recommended as these are considered the gold standard for patients who can assess and communicate their own pain.
- Use in accordance with local Trust policy.

  Common scales are:

- Numerical Pain Rating Scale (Williamson and Hoggart 2005) (Figure 20.1)
- Visual Analogue Scale (Gould et al. 2001) (Figure 20.2)
- Verbal Rating Scale (Jensen and Karoly 2011) (Figure 20.3).
- Wong–Baker Faces (Wong and Baker 1988) (Figure 20.4) can be used in those who can self-assess but have limited communication.

Procedure – Self-Assessment Scale

- Explain the procedure and scoring system.
- Ask the patient to score their pain.
- Consider analgesics, as required medication should be prescribed for those who score moderate to severe.
- Document the score.
- Escalate as appropriate.
- This type of pain assessment can be combined with the person's description of the location and quality of pain to gain a broader understanding of the pain and the interventions that may help (Table 20.1).

- When giving analgesia rescore the patient after adequate time has been given for therapeutic effect. A pain assessment is of little value without reassessment.

Procedure – PQRST Pain Assessment

- When pain is cardiac in nature, use PQRST to assess pain characteristics (Rogers et al. 1989) (Table 20.1).
- If severity can not be assessed, look for physiological and behavioural signs such as those in the Pain Assessment in Advanced Dementia (PAINAD) score (Table 20.3).

  NB: The acronym SOCRATES (Table 20.2; Clayton 2000) can also be used for assessing characteristics of pain.

Procedure – Assessing Pain in Individuals with Reduced Cognition

- Some scales, e.g. PAINAD (Warden et al. 2003) (Table 20.1) assess for pain in individuals with reduced cognition.
- Assess for five minutes and score each section:
  - Breathing.
  - Negative vocalisation.
  - Facial expression.
  - Body language.
  - Consolability.
- Each section scores between 0 and 2 to bring a total score out of 10.
- Document the score out of 10.
- Escalate appropriately.
- Carers can often provide insight into a person's usual behaviour and how they will express pain.

  NB: Where the behaviour of someone with a learning disability or dementia changes, pain should be considered as a possible cause

Red Flags

- ▶ Chest pain should be immediately investigated to rule out myocardial infarction.
- ▶ Causes of unexplained pain should always be investigated.
- ▶ Pain that is suggestive of nerve damage – often described as tingling or numb – should be urgently reviewed if it is unexplained.

References

Clayton, H.A, Reschak, G.L.C, Gaynor, S.E. & Creamer, J.L. (2000). A novel program to assess and manage pain. *MEDSURG Nursing.* 9 (6), 318–312.

Gould, D. et al. (2001). Visual analogue scale (VAS). *Journal of Clinical Nursing* 10: 697–706.

Jensen, M.P. and Karoly, P. (2011). Self-report scales and procedures for assessing pain in adults. In: *Handbook of Pain Assessment*, 3e (eds. D.C. Turk and R. Melzack), 19–44. New York: Guilford Press.

McCaffery, M. (1968). *Nursing Practice Theories Related to Cognition, Bodily Pain, and Man-Environment Interactions.* Los Angeles: University of California.

Rogers, J., Osborn, H., and Pousada, L. (1989). *Emergency Nursing: A Practical Guide.* Baltimore: Williams & Wilkins.

Warden, V., Hurley, A.C., and Volicer, L. (2003). Development and psychometric evaluation of the pain assessment in advanced dementia (PAINAD) scale. *Journal of the American Medical Directors Association* 4 (1): 9–15.

Williamson, A. and Hoggart, B. (2005). Pain: a review of three commonly used pain rating scales. *Journal of Clinical Nursing* 14 (7): 798–804.

Wong, D.L. and Baker, C.M. (1988). Pain assessment in children: comparision of assessment scales. *Paediatric Nursing* 14 (1): 9–17.

21 Neurovascular assessment

Figure 21.1 Assessment of neurovascular status.

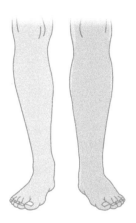

Changes in pulse, sensation and skin colour are late symptoms of neurovascular compromise (see front of chart for notes).	Neurovascular status	Pulse (with/without doppler)	Present	•										
			Reduced in volume or rate since last assessment												
			Not present												
		Sensation	Normal	•											
			Abnormal/has changed from last assessment												
		Skin colour	Normal, responsive capillary refill	•											
			Pallor and/or slow/absent capillary refill												

Any abnormal neurovascular status observations should be escalated immediately to the responsible clinician as per trust guidelines.

| | Initial | EX | | | | | | | | | | | | |

Figure 21.2 Pallor in limb.

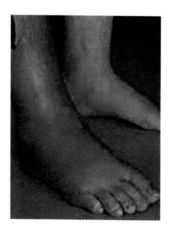

Figure 21.3 Passive movements.

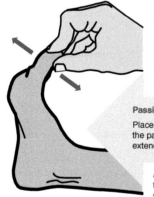

Passive movement of the fingers
Place your fingers underneath the patient's fingers and gently extend the fingers.

Passive movement of the toes
Place your fingers underneath the patient's toes and gently extend the toes.

An increase in pain when carrying out this test may indicate a developing compartment syndrome and should be recorded appropriately on the chart overleaf.

A second chart will be required to provide a minimum of 48 hours monitoring.

Table 21.1 Escalation of findings.

Pain	Severe and progressively worsening pain with passive movement suggests neurovascular impairment (Johnston-Walker and Hardcastle 2011) and must be acted upon immediately
Pallor	Whitening of the skin can indicate reduced arterial supply, whereas blue can indicate venous stasis
Pulse	Weak, thready or absent pulse, or a capillary refill time of more than three seconds, indicates reduced arterial supply. No pulse suggests acute compartment syndrome
Paraesthesia	Numbness or tingling may indicate nerve damage
Paralysis	Loss of movement may indicate nerve damage
Pressure	Note swelling of limb, tightening of skin that may be shiny and firm to touch (Parveen et al. 2014)

Figure 21.4 Oedema at the site of injury.

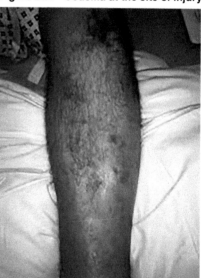

Clinical Nursing Skills at a Glance, First Edition. Edited by Sarah Curr and Carol Fordham-Clarke.
© 2022 John Wiley & Sons Ltd. Published 2022 by John Wiley & Sons Ltd.
Companion website: www.wiley.com/go/clinicalnursingskills

Background

- Neurovascular observations are carried out on at-risk limbs to detect early signs of acute compartment syndrome (ACS), which occurs when pressure increases in the body compartment, reducing blood supply to muscles and nerves.
- Damage can be permanent, so early detection is essential.
- Neurovascular assessment should be carried out after limb trauma, after application of an orthotic device, while a patient is in traction or plaster cast, and after surgery on a limb.
- Assessment considers circulation, sensory and motor function.
- Consider the six Ps (pain, pallor, pulse, paraesthesia, paralysis, and pressure) when assessing for ACS.

Influencing Factors

- Existing disabilities.
- Problems with communication.
- The unconscious patient.
- Unable or unwillingness to cooperate.
- Movement or access to pulse limited by plaster cast or orthotic device.

    Specific patients at risk are those with (RCN 2016):

- Orthopaedic injuries in those who are taking anticoagulants.
- High impact trauma.
- Crush injuries.
- Tibial, forearm, high impact distal fractures.

Professional Approach

- Obtain informed consent by ensuring the patient understands the assessment and why it is being performed.
- Ensure that you are both trained and competent to perform the assessment.
- Prior to completing the assessment, consider any interventions that may interfere with it, e.g. analgesia that masks pain.

Equipment

Use the neurovascular assessment chart of your local clinical area. Example of a chart is Figure 21.1.

Procedure

- Ensure that you follow the six Ps (Andrews 1990) for assessment of ACS:
  - Pain:
  - Undertake a full pain assessment (Chapter 20) and note any changes in characteristics and physiology of pain: is there pain in passive movement? Has the pain worsened?
  - Pallor:
    - Observe colour of skin, including the nail beds and internal mucosa.
    - Feel the warmth of the skin at site of injury and surrounding tissue.
    - If unsure, compare with the other limb (Figure 21.2).
    - Check capillary refill time (Chapter 36) to ascertain peripheral perfusion.
  - Pulse:
    - Check pulses that are situated distal to (away from) the site of concern.
    - Assess the pulse using the 0–4 system (Chapter 33).
    - Mark any pulses that are difficult to locate due to casts or traction.
  - Paraesthesia:
    - Check for limb sensation and note absence of sensation, numbness, tingling, or pins and needles.
  - Paralysis:
    - Check for paralysis by asking patient to move the peripherals, such as fingers and toes, related to the site of injury. If patient cannot move the site, move passively (Figure 21.3) and note any pain.
    - Check for range of motion and strength (Chapters 18, 20, and 52).
- Pressure:

    As ACS is increased pressure within a muscle where there is limited room for expansion (Parveen et al. 2014), noting any oedema present at the site of injury is also required (Figure 21.4).

- Post-assessment:
  - Document recordings and compare with last assessment and baseline.
  - Note changes of concern (Table 21.1) and escalate as appropriate, remembering that rapid reporting of changes can prevent permanent, irreversible, brain damage.
  - Reassess hourly for first 24 hours then 4-hourly for the next 24–48 hours (RCN 2016) in accordance with local Trust policy.

    NB: Remember that the highest risk of compartment syndrome is within 72 hours but can occur up to six days after the injury. Rapid detection and treatment of compartment syndrome can save a limb.

Red Flags

- Raised intracranial pressure.
- Absent pulses distal to site of injury.
- Cold, pale, limb.
- Inability to actively move muscle in the affected limb.

References

Andrews, L.W. (1990). Neurovascular assessment. *Advancing Clinical Care* 5 (6): 5–7.

Johnston-Walker, E. and Hardcastle, J. (2011). Neurovascular assessment in the critically ill patient. *Nursing in Critical Care* 16 (4): 170–177.

Parveen, A., Santy-Tomlinson, J., and Watson, R. (2014). Assessment and diagnosis of acute limb compartment syndrome: a literature review. *International Journal of Orthopaedic and Trauma Nursing* 18 (4): 180–190.

Royal College of Nursing (2016). *Peripheral Vascular Observation for Acute Limb Compartment Syndrome: RCN Consensus Guideline.* London: Royal College of Nursing.

22 Assessing and managing seizures

Figure 22.1 Tonic-clonic seizures.

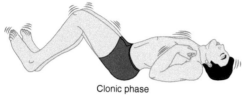

Tonic phase

Clonic phase

Figure 22.2 Atonic seizure.

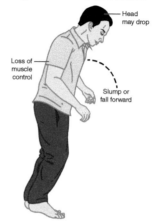

Head may drop

Loss of muscle control

Slump or fall forward

Figure 22.3 Focal seizures.

Automatisms

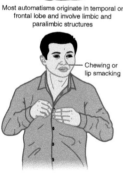

Most automatisms originate in temporal or frontal lobe and involve limbic and paralimbic structures

Chewing or lip smacking

Repetitive, seemingly purposeful activity such dressing and undressing or fumbling with buttons

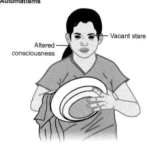

Altered consciousness

Vacant stare

Patient may unconsciously continue preictal activity

Hand clasping or rubbing

Pill-rolling movements

Figure 22.4 Absence seizures.

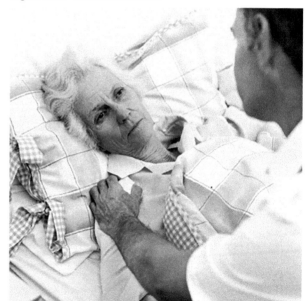

Table 22.1 Management and diagnosis following first seizure.

Management	Diagnosis
Essential health information education on how to recognise a seizure	Twelve-lead electrocardiogram on all adults
Details on immediate first aid during and after seizure for family and significant others	Routine blood tests to consider other causes/other comorbidities
Provide information on activities to be avoided during investigative stage, i.e. driving, lifting heavy equipment	Magnetic resonance imaging (MRI) is the imaging investigation of choice
Refer to epilepsy specialist	To be seen by a specialist for further investigations
NB: Make a neuropsychological referral in adults with educational or occupational challenges	NB: Only perform electroencephalogram to support epilepsy diagnosis

Source: Adapted from National Institute of Health and Care Excellence (2020).

Background

A seizure is increased electrical activity in the brain, sometimes described as a burst of activity, that interrupts normal brain function and can result in motor and sensory responses. Although people can have seizures for a variety of different reasons, they most commonly occur in epilepsy. A seizure can also occur as a result of alcohol withdrawal or in hypo- or hyperglycaemia, and once the underlying cause is treated the seizures will stop (NICE 2020).

Although epilepsy is often diagnosed in childhood, individuals can be diagnosed later in life following cerebrovascular accident or traumatic brain injury (NICE 2019). In infants, febrile seizures can also occur. It has been suggested that there are more than 40 different seizure presentations (Fisher et al. 2017), with the most common being:

- Generalised tonic-clonic (previously grand mal).
- Myoclonic.
- Tonic.
- Atonic.
- Focal (previously referred to as partial).
- Absences.

While generalised tonic-clonic (**GTC**) (Figure 22.1) is what most people consider a seizure due to loss of consciousness and jerking movements, not all seizures cause a loss of consciousness. A myoclonic seizure causes muscles to jerk, often after waking (Epilepsy Society 2020), a tonic seizure causes the person to become stiff and often fall over, whereas an atonic seizure causes the muscles to relax suddenly (Figure 22.2), usually resulting in the individual falling (Epilepsy Society 2020). Focal seizures can cause unusual sensations, such as numbness, tingling, or an unusual smell or taste but can also cause lip-smacking, pulling at clothes (Figure 22.3) as well as the more expected jerking movements (Epilepsy Society 2020). Absences, previously called petit mal, are non-motor seizures and result in the person becoming blank or unresponsive (Figure 22.4). All of these require immediate management as well as diagnostic tests (Table 22.1).

Influencing Factors

As highlighted above, seizures can be caused by chemical imbalances as well as other neurological conditions. In the person living with epilepsy, there are often triggers that can increase the likelihood of seizure occurrence. These could be (Epilepsy Action 2020):

- Not taking medication as prescribed.
- Altered sleep patterns.
- Altered mealtimes, eating habits.
- Stress.
- Alcohol or drug use.
- Hormonal changes, i.e. menstruation.
- Flashing or flickering lights.

Professional Approach

- Where possible, obtain a full history and establish if there are any triggers or warning signs.
- In the secondary care setting ensure intravenous access.
- Ask the patient how they manage their seizures and what usually helps.

Equipment – Managing all Seizures

- A fob watch or watch with a second hand.
- For GTC a cushion or pillow to protect the head and limbs is recommended.
- In status epilepticus, a prolonged or continuous seizures, high-flow oxygen is required.

Procedure – Generalised Tonic-Clonic Seizure

Use the ACTION mnemonic (Epilepsy Action 2018):

A – *Assess*. For safety, this may involve lowering the bed to the floor, loosening clothing if necessary.

C – *Cushion*. This will generally involve placing a cushion under the head but may also involve padding the bed sides to prevent injury to the limbs.

T – *Time*. Start timing as soon as the seizure starts.

I – *Identify*. In the out-of-hospital setting look for a medical bracelet and other information. In the care setting, ascertain if there is intravenous access and what medication has been prescribed.

O – *Over*. Once the seizure has stopped roll the person over into the recovery position (Chapter 12), ensuring that the airway is protected.

N – *Never* restrain or try to move the person, as this can cause more harm.

NB: If someone is in a wheelchair, leave them, where possible, as moving could cause further injury.

Procedure – Status Epilepticus

In the out-of-hospital setting an ambulance will need to be called. In the in hospital setting, specific guidance is given for the status epilepticus (NICE 2020):

- First stage – secure airway:
  - Administer high-flow oxygen.
  - Assess cardiorespiratory function.
  - Ensure intravenous access.
- Second stage – monitor.

NB: If unresolved after treatment consider intubation and intensive care unit admission.

Procedure – Focal Seizures and Absences

- Time the event.
- Guide the person away from danger.
- Stay until the person is fully recovered.
- Be calm and reassuring, and when the person is ready let them know what happened.

Red Flags

- Status epilepticus is an emergency and requires immediate first aid and hospital admission.
- Complaint of a thunderclap or intense headache prior to seizure could indicate subarachnoid haemorrhage, an emergency requiring immediate hospital treatment and management.

References

Epilepsy Action (2018) *First Aid for Epileptic Seizures*. www.epilepsy. org.uk/sites/epilepsy/files/info/first-aid-seizures-poster.jpg (accessed 28 October 2020).

Epilepsy Action (2020) *Seizure Triggers*. www.epilepsy.org.uk/info/ triggers?utm_source=Gads&utm_medium=CPC&utm_ campaign=AITriggers&utm_content=&gclid=CjwKCAjw8-78BRA 0EiwAFUw8LDhhho7174Cf3h5Blt9yHwhi7KM7Wo94819B34w3s fCHJ03-KEfQaxoCjacQAvD_BwE (accessed 28 October 2020).

Epilepsy Society (2020) *Seizure Types*. www.epilepsysociety.org.uk/ seizure-types?gclid=CjwKCAjw8-78BRA0EiwAFUw8LLUfiHjh0Fxj- AYulm4Q7-QKsezUXcv2mtWzaTI3dN_8i_u4H8_ANBo C3KQQAvD_BwE (accessed 28 October 2020).

Fisher, R.S., Cross, H., French, J.A. et al. (2017). Operational classification of seizure types by the international league against epilepsy: position paper of the ILAE commission for classification and terminology. *Epilepsia* 58 (4): 522–530.

National Institute for Health and Care Excellence (2019) *Epilepsy: What else might it be?* https://cks.nice.org.uk/topics/epilepsy/ diagnosis/differential-diagnosis (accessed 28 October 2020).

National Institute for Health and Care Excellence (2020). *CG 137 Epilepsy Diagnosis & Management*. London: National Institute for Health and Care Excellence, London.

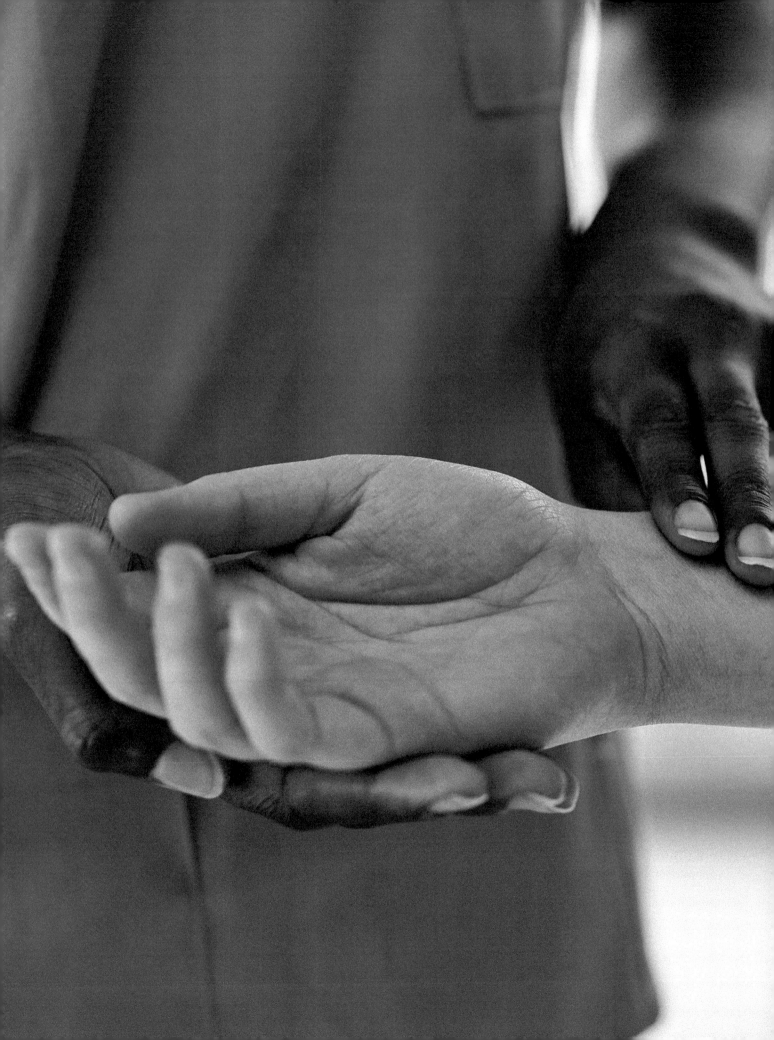

Respiratory skills

Part 5

Chapters

23 Assessing and managing the airway

Figure 23.1 Tongue obstructing the airway.

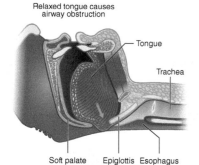

Relaxed tongue causes airway obstruction

Tongue

Trachea

Soft palate   Epiglottis   Esophagus

Figure 23.3 (a) Nasopharyngeal airways. (b) Measuring for the correct size.

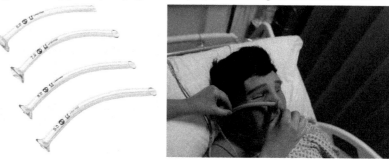

Figure 23.2 Suction equipment.

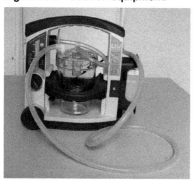

Figure 23.4 Oropharyngeal airways.

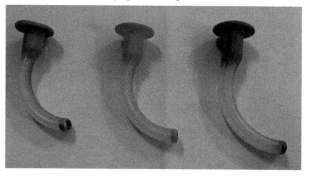

Figure 23.5 Oropharyngeal airways: (a) measurement; (b) insertion (*Source*: Redrawn from Resuscitation Guidelines, 2016).

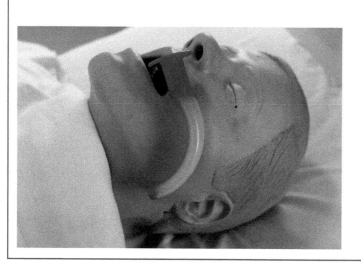

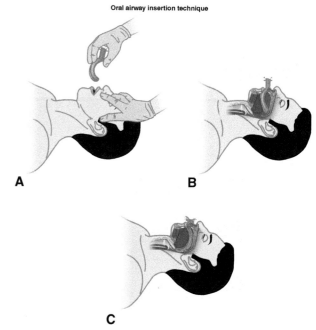

Oral airway insertion technique

A

B

C

Background

In the acutely unwell adult an ABCDE approach to assessment is recommended (NICE 2007) and, as such, in any assessment it is essential to establish whether the airway is patent. A patent airway is one that is open and clear of obstruction.

It is important to note that any obstruction of the airway is a clinical emergency and should be addressed immediately. In some instances, the airway obstruction may be remedied by a head tilt/chin lift and use of the recovery position, whereas in other circumstances advanced airway management may be required.

Influencing Factors

The airway can be obstructed by:

- Secretions.
- Blood.
- Vomit.
- Teeth.
- Tumours.
- Swelling, such as in anaphylaxis.
- The tongue.

NB: A reduction in consciousness can lead to an unprotected airway and the tongue will obstruct the airway if the patient is unconscious and lying on their back (Figure 23.1).

Professional Approach

- Ensure that you explain what you are doing and why, in order to reassure the patient.
- Work within your level of training and competence and call for more advanced help and expert advice as required.

Equipment

Equipment may include:

- Suction.
- Nasopharyngeal airways.
- Oropharyngeal airways.
- Cardiac Arrest trolley for other airway adjuncts.

Procedure – Assessing the Airway

Begin by establishing whether the patient is responsive and therefore able to maintain their own airway. If the patient can talk, the airway is patent.

NB: If the patient is unresponsive, they may not be able to protect their airway

- *Complete airway obstruction* – no movement of air is present at the mouth, nothing is heard or felt. Use of accessory muscles and paradoxical breathing may be seen (the chest moves inwards during inhalation and not outwards as normal)
- *Partial airway obstruction* – air is detected at the mouth and breathing is noisy. Noises heard are likened to grunting, gurgling or snoring.

- *Stridor* – obstruction at the larynx or above causing a high-pitched vibrating sound. Snoring is often heard when the tongue occludes the pharynx.

> Obtain immediate help if the airway is partially or fully obstructed

Procedure – Managing the Airway

- Suction – use a Yankauer sucker to remove blood, vomit, and other secretions (Figure 23.2).
- If the patient is unconscious use the head tilt/chin lift manoeuvre to prevent the tongue from obstructing the airway (Figure 11.1)
- The following airway adjuncts could be used to maintain a patent airway;
- Nasopharyngeal airways (Figure 23.3a) can be used on patients who are semi-conscious or unconscious. Size is determined by measuring from the edge of the nose to the tragus of the ear (Figure 23.3b) – use the largest diameter size that fits easily into the nostril.
- Oropharyngeal airways (Figure 23.4) will only be tolerated by unconscious patients where the gag reflex is lost. To ensure the correct size is used, measure from the incisor to the angle of the jaw (Figure 23.5a) (Resuscitation Council UK 2016).

Procedure – Inserting an Oropharyngeal Airway

- Apply non-sterile gloves.
- Measure the correct size.
- Open the patient's mouth to check that it is free from any secretions.
- Suction mouth if necessary.
- Initially insert airway into mouth "upside down" and then rotate 180° to prevent pushing tongue (Figure 23.5b) backwards and obstructing airway (Resuscitation Council UK 2016)
- Check that the patient is breathing.
- Remove gloves and decontaminate hands.

Red Flags

- Airway obstruction is a medical emergency.
- It is essential to be able to recognise the first signs of airway obstruction.
- Nasopharyngeal airways must never be inserted in patients with facial injuries, severe head injuries, or basal skull fractures.
- A patient with a compromised airway will require oxygen.

References

National Institute of Health and Care Excellence (2007). *CG50 Acutely Ill Adults in Hospital: Recognising and Responding to Deterioration*. London: National Institute of Health and Care Excellence.

Resuscitation Council UK (2016). *Resuscitation Guidelines*. London: Resuscitation Council.

24 Respiratory assessment

Figure 24.1 Inhalation and exhalation.

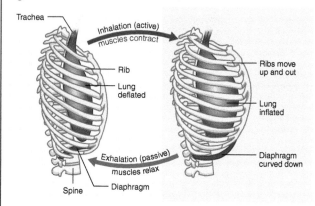

Table 24.1 Sputum assessment.

Quality of sputum	Indication
Clear	Normal mucus
White	Asthma/chronic obstructive pulmonary disease
White/frothy (may be bloodstained)	Pulmonary oedema
Yellow/green	Infection
Blood in sputum (haemoptysis)	Possible lung cancer, tuberculosis, pulmonary embolism, pneumonia
Foul odour	Lung abscess

Table 24.2 Respiratory rates (RCP 2017).

Rate	Definition
Normal	14–20 breaths/minute
Tachypnoea	> 20 breaths/minute
Bradypnoea	< 8 breaths/minute

Table 24.3 Abnormal effort in breathing.

Effort	Description
Normal	Chest expands on inhalation, both sides of the chest expand equally, breathing is relaxed, quiet and automatic
Dyspnoea	Breathlessness and discomfort with breathing
Exertional dyspnoea	Shortness of breath on exercise
Orthopnoea	Shortness of breath lying down
Paroxysmal nocturnal dyspnoea	Sudden breathlessness that occurs at night when the patient is lying flat
Paroxysmal breathing	Chest wall moves inward on inhalation, expanding on exhalation

Table 24.4 Abnormal patterns of breathing.

Pattern	Description
Kussmaul respirations	Fast and deep respiration, seen in metabolic acidosis
Apnoeustic respiration	Prolonged gasping during inspiration followed by short expiration, seen in lesions affecting the pons
Agonal (previously Cheyne–Stokes)	Episodes of increasing depth of respiration followed by decrease, resulting in apnoea

Clinical Nursing Skills at a Glance, First Edition. Edited by Sarah Curr and Carol Fordham-Clarke.
© 2022 John Wiley & Sons Ltd. Published 2022 by John Wiley & Sons Ltd.
Companion website: www.wiley.com/go/clinicalnursingskills

Background

Breathing is controlled by the autonomic nervous system which means that we do not have to think about our breathing usually, but we will be aware that we are breathing faster when exerting ourselves and slower at rest. Breathing consists of both inhalation and exhalation, with inhalation bringing in oxygen from the air and exhalation removing carbon dioxide, the waste product of cellular respiration.

In humans inhalation occurs when the pressure in the lungs drops below that of atmospheric pressure. We then inhale to equalise the pressure and this inhalation requires the volume of the thoracic cavity to be increased. This is achieved by the diaphragm and intercostal muscles contracting as a result of nervous stimulation from the respiratory centres in the medulla oblongata, in the brain stem (Marieb and Hoehn 2018). Exhalation then occurs when the muscles relax as the lung volume decreases, causing high pressure, which exhalation then remedies (Figure 24.1).

Influencing Factors

When breathing is laboured, a visual respiratory assessment is required. This includes inspection of the chest, face, and peripheries, as well as assessment of respiratory rate, depth, and pattern. The indications for undertaking a respiratory assessment are:

- To obtain a baseline of the patient's respiratory rate for comparison with future respiratory rates.
- To monitor any changes in the patient's respiratory status.
- To ensure prompt and appropriate interventions.
- To evaluate responses to treatments that support breathing and influence the respiratory system.

NB: If any results are abnormal then a senior healthcare professional must be informed.

Professional Approach

- Always explain what you are doing and why, in order to obtain informed consent and reassure the patient.
- Remember that only a trained and competent person can perform this assessment.

Equipment

A fob watch, or watch with second hand.

Procedure – Inspection

The following areas should be assessed;

- The patient's general appearance. Is the patient exhausted? Is the patient emaciated? Is the patient in pain?
- Skin colour. Is the patient pale (possible anaemia)? Is there a bluish tinge around the lips or peripherally? This is termed cyanosis and indicates a lack of oxygen.
- Use of accessory muscles in the neck, back, and abdomen to assist ventilation.
- The shape of chest.
- Any scars on the chest.
- Chest wall movement – is it equal?
- Audible breath sounds, e.g. a wheeze. When does it occur?
- Observe for signs of increased effort in breathing, such as nasal flaring, pursed lips, gasping, and accessory muscle usage (muscles of neck, shoulders and abdomen).
- Does the patient have a cough? Is it productive?
- Is the patient able to hold a conversation?

Procedure – Sputum Assessment

Observe a cough for:

- Strength.
- Dryness.
- Wetness.
- Hoarseness.
- Frequency.

If the patient coughs up sputum (expectorates) it is important to observe the:

- Colour.
- Consistency.
- Quality.
- Odour (Table 24.1).

Procedure – Assessing Respirations

Respirations are observed for the rate, depth, and pattern of the patient's breathing.

Rate

- Use fob watch and count for one minute.
- To ensure accuracy of the observation it is better if the patient is unaware that the respiration rate is being counted. This can be undertaken directly after taking the patient's pulse (Table 24.2).

Depth

- Assess the depth of chest expansion which equates to the volume of air moving in and out in one breath.
- Observe for any signs of distress or alteration from the normal breathing pattern (Table 24.3).

Pattern

- Assess the pattern of respirations to see if they are regular, irregular, deep, or shallow (Table 24.4).
- Can the patient hold a conversation or are they focused on breathing?

Pain

If the patient complains of pain, identify the type of pain and if it is related to inhalation or exhalation.

Red Flags

- Cyanosis is a late sign of poor oxygenation and suggests that the person is critically ill. This requires emergency oxygen administration (O'Driscoll et al. 2017), immediate escalation of care, and full vital signs monitoring.
- While visual signs of increased respiratory effort require escalation of care, a silent, non-moving chest, despite effort, is a medical emergency.
- Breathing that is irregular and inconsistent could be agonal breathing. This is incompatible with life.

References

Marieb, E.N. and Hoehn, K. (2018). *Human Anatomy & Physiology*, 11e. Pearsons: Harlow.

O'Driscoll, B.R., Howard, L., Earis, J. et al. (2017). BTS guideline for oxygen for oxygen use in adults in healthcare and emergency settings. *Thorax* 72 (1): i1–i188.

Royal College of Physicians (2017). *National Early Warning Score (NEWS) 2: Standardising the Assessment of Acute Illness Severity in the NHS. Report of a Working Party*. Royal College of Physicians: London.

25 Monitoring oxygen saturations

Figure 25.1   Peripheral O₂ monitoring.

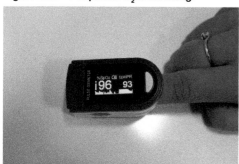

Figure 25.2   (a) Ear O₂ monitoring. (b) Nasal O₂ monitoring.

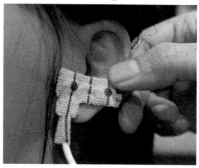
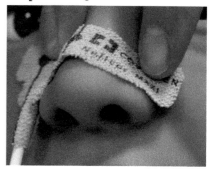

Figure 25.3   National Early Warning Score (NEWS) scoring: SpO₂ levels and O₂ administration.

A+B Respirations Breaths/min													
	≥25												
	21–24												2
	18–20												
	15–17												
	12–14												
	9–11												1
	≤8												3
A+B SpO₂ Scale 1 Oxygen saturation (%)	≥96												
	94–95												1
	92–93												2
	≤91												3
SpO₂ Scale 2† Oxygen saturation (%)	≥97 on O₂												3
Use Scale 2 if target range is 88–92%, eg in hypercapnic respiratory failure	95–96 on O₂												2
	93–94 on O₂												1
	≥93 on air												
	88–92												
†ONLY use Scale 2 under the direction of a qualified clinician	86–87												1
	84–85												2
	≤83%												3
Air or oxygen?	A=Air												
	O₂ L/min												
	Device												2

Clinical Nursing Skills at a Glance, First Edition. Edited by Sarah Curr and Carol Fordham-Clarke.
© 2022 John Wiley & Sons Ltd. Published 2022 by John Wiley & Sons Ltd.
Companion website: www.wiley.com/go/clinicalnursingskills

Background

Oxygen combines with the haemoglobin molecules within the red blood cells in the lungs in order to be carried to the tissues where it is released. Every haemoglobin molecule can combine with up to four molecules of oxygen, where it becomes saturated, and this combination of haemoglobin and oxygen is labelled oxyhaemoglobin.

This saturation of haemoglobin by oxygen is measured by the pulse oximetry probe. This painless, inexpensive, non-invasive method can be easily placed on the finger and allows for continued monitoring. The two-sided device works on the principle that blood saturated with oxygen is a different colour from blood depleted of oxygen and thus the infrared light that it emits is absorbed differently depending on whether the haemoglobin is saturated or not (Myatt 2017). The resulting reading denotes peripheral oxygen saturation, commonly referred to as SpO_2, and this is registered as a percentage (Figure 25.1).

Pulse oximetry is usually measured peripherally on the finger but can also be placed on the earlobe or taped to the bridge of the nose (Myatt 2017) (Figure 25.2). Fundamentally it is indicated in any clinical situation where hypoxaemia is likely to occur, such as:

- During oxygen therapy to monitor effect.
- If the patient becomes clinically unstable, e.g. fall in blood pressure.
- If the patient is sedated.
- During anaesthesia.
- In exacerbation of respiratory conditions such as chronic obstructive pulmonary disease (COPD) or asthma.

Influencing Factors

- Peripheral vasoconstriction and poor peripheral circulation will result in reduced pulse detection and inaccurate measurement of oxygen saturation levels.
- Cardiac dysrhythmias, e.g. atrial fibrillation, can cause poor peripheral perfusion, resulting in a falsely low reading.
- Inflating the blood pressure cuff on the arm where the probe is placed will interrupt the ability of the pulse oximeter to read the oxygen level.
- Patient movement i.e. shivering, tremors.
- Nail varnish (dark colours) and false nails will cause an inaccurate reading.
- Bright or fluorescent room lights may interfere with light transmission on the probe.

Professional Approach

- Ensure that the probe is fully functionally before approaching the patient.
- Explain why the measurement is being recorded to obtain informed consent.
- If nail varnish is to be removed, provide a sound rationale for this to the patient.
- Depending on the patient's condition a peripheral measurement may not be appropriate, and an appropriate probe should be used to monitor central oxygen saturation (Figure 25.2).

- The healthcare professional must be competent at performing the procedure but also at recognising what the reading indicates. As such, an awareness of the normal oxygen saturation range, between 95% and 100%, and ranges that may be normal for other client groups, such as those with COPD having a range of 88–92% (O'Driscoll et al. 2017), is vital, as well as the knowledge of when to escalate care.

Equipment

- Appropriate pulse oximetry probe for site.
- Access to hand decontaminant.
- Nail varnish remover (as required).

Procedure

- Switch the probe on to ensure it is functioning effectively and emitting an infrared light.
- Check that the oximeter is also displaying a waveform or bar graph. This demonstrates that a pulse is detected.
- Set alarm limits.
- Clean with a hard surface wipe, in accordance with manufacturer's guidance and local policy.
- Approach the patient and introduce yourself, then provide an explanation and rationale to obtain informed consent.
- Decontaminate hands.
- Assess for any factors that may affect the accuracy of the reading.
- Ensure the patient's skin is clean, dry and warm.
- Remove the patient's nail polish/false nails.
- Place the probe on the selected finger.
- If the oxygen saturation is to be measured continuously, note the site and time the probe is placed. Make sure the probe is observed at every patient contact point and moved to another digit every two hours (Gefen et al. 2020).
- Document the reading, noting if oxygen is being administered (Figure 25.3).
- Report any changes or abnormalities and escalate as appropriate, in accordance with National Early Warning Score (NEWS) 2.
- Clean the machine and store correctly.
- Decontaminate hands.
- Ensure the patient is left comfortable.

Red Flags

- ☛ Carbon monoxide poisoning can present with a normal SpO_2.
- ☛ Below 85% the oxygen saturation reading is not accurate and requires escalation and potentially an arterial blood gas.

References

Gefen, A., Alves, P., Ciprandi, G. et al. (2020). Device-related pressure ulcers: SECURE prevention. *Journal of Wound Care* 29 (Sup2a): S1–S52.

Myatt, R. (2017). Pulse oximetry: what the nurse needs to know. *Nursing Standard* 31 (31): 42–45.

O'Driscoll, B.R., Howard, L., Earis, J. et al. (2017). BTS guideline for oxygen for oxygen use in adults in healthcare and emergency settings. *Thorax* 72 (1): i1–i188.

26 Arterial blood gas analysis

Table 26.1 Situations where arterial blood gases (ABGs) should be measured.

* All critically ill patients or those at risk of deterioration
* Unexpected hypoxaemia (SaO_2 < 94%)
* Deteriorating SaO_2 in a patient with previously stable hypoxaemia, e.g. COPD
* A patient requiring supplementary oxygen to achieve target saturations
* A previously stable patient requiring increased oxygen administration
* Patients with risk factors for hypercapnic respiratory failure, increased breathlessness, decreasing SaO_2 or drowsiness or other symptoms of CO_2 retention
* Breathless patients at risk of metabolic conditions, e.g. diabetic ketoacidosis
* Post-cardiorespiratory arrest
* Evaluation of intervention impact such as oxygen therapy, or respiratory support

Source: O'Driscoll et al. (2017).

Table 26.2 Arterial blood gas (ABG) interpretation.

Parameter	Normal value	Indications of abnormalities
pH	7.35–7.45	> 7.45 is alkalosis and < 7.35 is acidosis. Changes in pH may reflect respiratory or metabolic causes and therefore it is necessary to examine $PaCO_2$ (respiratory) and HCO_3 (metabolic) which act as buffers to keep pH within the required range
Partial pressure of carbon dioxide – $PaCO_2$	4.5–6.0 kPa	> 6.0 kPa is respiratory acidosis and < 4.5 kPa is respiratory alkalosis
Partial pressure of oxygen – PaO_2	11.5–13 kPa	< 11.5 is a low partial pressure which could be caused by obstruction, reducing oxygen intake or hypoventilation > 13 is high partial pressure which could be caused by pulmonary oedema or lung disease
Bicarbonate – HCO_3	22–26 mmol/L	> 26 is metabolic alkalosis and < 22 is metabolic acidosis
Base excess (BE)	–2 to +2 mmol/L	A BE > –2 is low, indicative of a metabolic acidosis. A high BE, > 2+, could indicate a metabolic alkalosis
Arterial oxygen saturation – SaO_2	94–98%	This is often monitored non-invasively

Source: Adapted from Gibson (2017).

Figure 26.1 Arterial line setup.

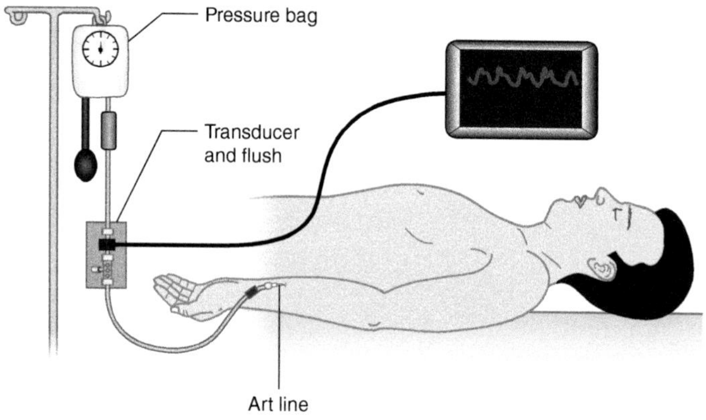

Pressure bag
Transducer and flush
Art line

Figure 26.2 Arterial blood gas (ABG) wave formation.

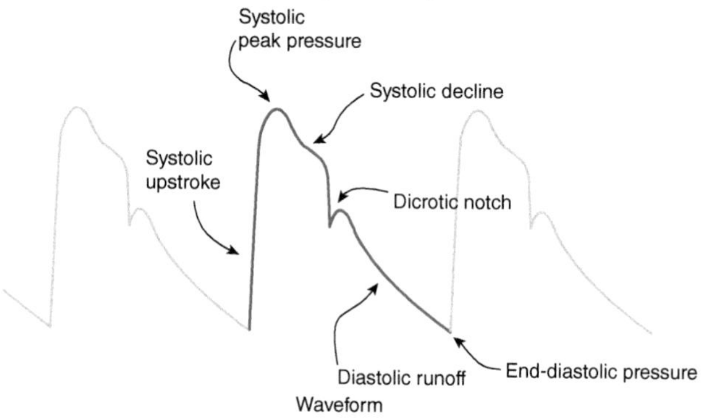

Systolic peak pressure
Systolic decline
Systolic upstroke
Dicrotic notch
Diastolic runoff
End-diastolic pressure
Waveform

Clinical Nursing Skills at a Glance, First Edition. Edited by Sarah Curr and Carol Fordham-Clarke.
© 2022 John Wiley & Sons Ltd. Published 2022 by John Wiley & Sons Ltd.
Companion website: www.wiley.com/go/clinicalnursingskills

Background

Arterial blood gas interpretation provides information on the quality of pulmonary gas exchange, and acid–base balance and is an essential part of diagnosing and managing a patient's respiratory and metabolic status. In this way it assesses the ability of the patient to maintain normal cellular function as ostensibly small changes in pH can have significant effects on the body. As such arterial blood gas (ABG) sampling and interpretation are common requirements in healthcare.

Influencing Factors

- Situations where ABGs may need to be taken and analysed are shown in Table 26.1.
- In order to measure an ABG the healthcare professional needs to be aware of the normal parameters, outlined in Table 26.2.

Professional Approach

- The correct interpretation of ABGs will require additional knowledge of the patient, such as their medical history, a full clinical assessment and comparison with previous ABG readings or the patient's norm.
- Any abnormalities detected must be promptly communicated to the multidisciplinary team and acted upon.
- Prior to ABG sampling explain procedure and rationale.

Equipment

- Tray to hold sampling equipment.
- 5 mL syringe.
- ABG heparinised sampling syringe.
- 70% isopropyl alcohol and 2% chlorhexidine impregnated wipe (for port cleansing).
- Non-sterile gloves and disposable apron.
- Appropriate documentation charts.

Procedure – ABG Sampling

As an ABG is obtained from a direct arterial puncture or an arterial line, often in the radial artery, it must only be obtained by a skilled and suitably qualified practitioner. Although sampling from an arterial line is more common, the below procedure must only be performed by those trained and deemed competent in ABG sampling:

- Gather equipment and approach the patient.
- Check the fluid bag and giving set for patency.
- Check the pressure bag remains at 300 mmHg.
- Check that the transducer is at the phlebostatic axis (Figure 26.1).
- Check the site and dressing using the VIP score (Chapter 71).
- Check the wave formation (Figure 26.2).
- Prepare equipment.
- Decontaminate hands and put on gloves and apron.
- Cleanse port for 30 seconds, allowing to dry for a further 30 seconds (Loveday et al. 2014).
- Attach the 5 mL syringe.
- Turn the three-way tap off to fluids and on to the patient.
- Remove 5 mL of blood.
- Turn the three-way tap back to first position.
- Remove syringe.
- Attach ABG sampling syringe and turn three-way tap off to fluids and on to patient.
- Remove 1 mL.
- Turn the three-way tap back to first position.
- Remove syringe ensuring excess air is expelled.
- Ensure a healthcare professional trained in its use takes the sample to the blood sampling machine.
- Operate the flush system to clear the line of blood.
- Analyse sample as outlined below.

Procedure – ABG Analysis

- There are three main groups of results to be analysed from the arterial blood sample:
  - pH.
  - respiratory function (oxygen, carbon dioxide, saturation).
  - metabolic measures (bicarbonate, base excess).
- Carry out the analysis of the ABG systematically.
- First assess the level of oxygenation by examining the partial pressure of oxygen (PaO_2), arterial oxygen saturation (SaO_2) and haemoglobin. As normal PaO_2 is 11.5–13 kPa, decide if the PaO_2 indicates hypoxaemia.
- Type 1 respiratory failure involves hypoxaemia ($PaO_2 < 8$ kPa) with normocapnia ($PaCO_2 < 6.0$ kPa).
- Type 2 respiratory failure involves hypoxaemia ($PaO_2 < 8$ kPa) with hypercapnia ($PaCO_2 > 6.0$ kPa).
- Next determine if the pH level is within the normal parameters of 7.35–7.45. In acidosis the pH is < 7.35. In alkalosis the pH is > 7.45.
- Assess the respiratory component by examining the $PaCO_2$ with normocapnia in the range 4.5–6.0 kPa. A $PaCO_2 > 6.0$ kPa coupled with a low pH indicates a respiratory acidosis. A $PaCO_2 < 4.5$ kPa coupled with a high pH indicates a respiratory alkalosis.
- Next assess the metabolic component by determining if bicarbonate (HCO_3) is within normal limits. If $HCO_3 < 22$ together with a low pH, this is indicative of metabolic acidosis. An $HCO_3 > 26$ together with a high pH indicates a metabolic alkalosis.
- Document results and escalate care as appropriate.

Examination of the pH will show if compensation has taken place. In compensation, the body attempts to respond to an acid–base disorder to stabilize pH, either by excretion via the kidneys, or retention or excretion of CO_2 via the lungs. Therefore, pH is normal but $PaCO_2$ and HCO_3 are abnormal.

Red Flags

- The haemoglobin content will affect the ability to transport oxygen, thereby affecting PaO_2 and SaO_2 levels.
- If PaO_2 and SaO_2 levels are higher than normal, this may indicate unnecessarily high levels of supplementary oxygen administration.
- A normal pH does not exclude respiratory or metabolic pathology. Ensure all values are systematically analysed.
- PaO_2 and SaO_2 must always be interpreted with regard to supplementary oxygen being administered and haemoglobin level.

References

Gibson, V. (2017). Pulse oximetry and arterial blood gas analysis. In: *Respiratory Care* (eds. V. Gibson and D. Waters). Boca Raton: CRC Press.

Loveday, H., Wilson, J.A., Pratt, R. et al. (2014). epic3: National Evidence-Based Guidelines for preventing healthcare-associated infections in NHS hospitals in England. *Journal of Hospital Infection* 86: S1–S70.

O'Driscoll, B.R., Howard, L.S., Earis, J., Mak, V. (2017) BTS guideline for oxygen use in adults in healthcare and emergency settings. *Thorax* 72: ii1–ii90.

27 Chest auscultation

Figure 27.1 Auscultation step ladder approach.

Auscultation

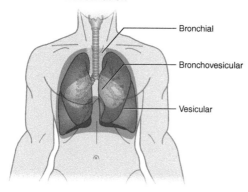

- Bronchial
- Bronchovesicular
- Vesicular

Figure 27.2 (a) Anterior position; (b) posterior position.

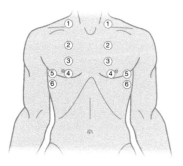

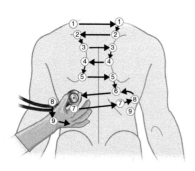

Table 27.1 Normal breath sounds. Note that the pitch of sounds is dependent upon area of lungs listened to.

Name	Location	Pitch
Bronchial	Trachea and main bronchi	High pitch and loud
Bronchovesicular	Between main bronchi and small airways	Medium pitch
Vesicular	Small, peripheral airways	Low pitch and faint

Source: Adapted from Sarkar et al. 2015.

Table 27.2 Abnormal breath sounds.

Name	Location	Sound
Crackles	Heard on inspiration and expiration when the airways that have been collapsed or blocked crack open	A "popping" sound. Due to secretions, e.g. sputum of fluid
Wheeze	Heard on expiration	Musical of high/low pitch. Caused by bronchospasm
Pleural rub	Heard on inspiration and expiration	Sound like creaking leather/walking in snow. Caused by inflammation of the pleural membranes
Stridor	Heard at the end of inspiration	Harsh high-pitched sound. Indicating laryngeal/tracheal obstruction
Bronchial	Normally heard over trachea and right and left main bronchi but can be heard anywhere	High pitch. Can be heard anywhere where there is consolidated lung tissue and where no gaseous exchange is taking, e.g. pneumonia

Source: Adapted from Sarkar et al. (2015).

Figure 27.3 Lateral position.

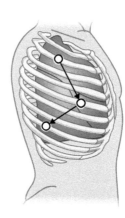

Background

Auscultation is a simple, non-invasive, easy-to-perform method for listening to breath sounds using a stethoscope (Sarkar et al. 2015). This is now taught at the pre-registration level in nursing (Nursing & Midwifery Council 2018) but competency will be acquired through working with a member of staff trained in this skill. As this identification and interpretation of sounds within the lungs form part of a holistic respiratory assessment, it can be undertaken by doctors, nurses, physiotherapists, and other competent healthcare professionals.

When performing auscultation, a systematic approach must be performed to ensure accurate interpretation of breath sounds and accurate description of the location of abnormal sounds. During this skill the breath sounds are auscultated over the anterior, posterior, and lateral chest wall surfaces (Coviello 2014).

Influencing Factors

- Environment – where possible choose a quiet environment free from external noise.
- Chaperone – the option of a chaperone or practitioner of the same gender may be preferred by some patients.
- Competency – in order to be competent in detection of abnormal breath sounds, it is necessary to be familiar with normal breath sounds at specific locations within the chest (Proctor and Rickards 2020) and to regularly perform this skill.
- Starting auscultation at the lung bases may be considered in older people, or those patients presenting with breathlessness.
- If the patient cannot adopt a sitting posture, ask/assist them to roll laterally to examine the back.
- Excessive fat or shallow breathing may affect the clarity of breath sounds.

Professional Approach

- Provide explanations and obtain informed consent.
- Follow local policy for decontamination and infection control.
- Maintain privacy, dignity, and comfort.
- Ensure that the stethoscope is fully functioning and that you have competency in stethoscope use and interpreting sounds.
- If you feel the patient is too unwell for assessment and requires immediate management, provide treatment as able. Remember that high-flow oxygen can be given by all registered staff in an emergency (O'Driscoll et al. 2017) and escalate immediately to senior staff and appropriate members of the multidisciplinary team.

Equipment

- Stethoscope with diaphragm locked into position.
- Single-use decontamination swab (impregnated with 70% alcohol or 2% chlorhexidine in 70% alcohol in accordance with local Trust policy).

Procedure

- Introduce yourself, confirm patient identification, explain procedure, and obtain informed consent.
- Ensure that the patient is in an appropriate position, preferably sitting upright, or leaning slightly forwards.
- Close the curtains or door to maintain privacy and dignity while also minimising disturbances.
- Decontaminate hands and equipment.
- Insert stethoscope earpieces facing forward towards the nose, creating a seal to reduce external noise.
- Place diaphragm of the stethoscope on the anterior chest using gentle pressure.
- Ask the patient to take a breath in and out through an open mouth.
- Auscultating from side-to-side and top-to-bottom (i.e. a step ladder approach), listen between the intercostal spaces to the breath sounds for a full respiratory cycle. (Figure 27.1).
- Listen for the quality and intensity of the breath sounds, and the presence of adventitious sounds (Tables 27.1 and 27.2).
- Systematically compare the opposite sides of the chest, listening for asymmetry (Figure 27.2).
- Apply the same method to the posterior chest while avoiding listening over the scapulae.
- Asking the patient to move their right arm, listen to the right lateral chest (the three lobes of the right lung) (Figure 27.3), then in the left lateral position listen to the upper and lower lobes.
- Once completed, assist the patient to dress if required and ensure comfort.
- Discuss your findings with the patient and respond to any questions.
- Decontaminate hands and equipment.
- Inform the senior nurse/appropriate member of the medical team of the findings.
- Document the findings in the patient's notes, noting the location and quality of the sounds. This documentation includes normal breath sounds, reduced or abnormal breath sounds, and absent breath sounds.

Red Flags

- When auscultating do not listen over the bone but in the spaces between the ribs, the intercostal spaces (Proctor and Rickards 2020), to ensure accuracy of findings.
- Absence of breath sounds may indicate pneumothorax, pleural effusion or lobar collapse.
- Do not apply too much pressure to the diaphragm, as this will filter out low-pitched sounds.
- Never listen through clothing, as this affects sound transmission.

References

Coviello, J.S. (2014). *Auscultation Skills: Breath and Heart Sounds*, 5e. Philadelphia: Wolters Kluwer.

Nursing & Midwifery Council (2018). *Future Nurse: Standards of Proficiency for Registered Nurses*. London: Nursing & Midwifery Council.

O'Driscoll, B.R., Howard, L., Earis, J. et al. (2017). BTS guideline for oxygen for oxygen use in adults in healthcare and emergency settings. *Thorax* 72 (1): i1–i188.

Proctor, J. and Rickards, E. (2020). How to perform chest auscultation and interpret the findings. *Nursing Times* 116 (1): 23–26.

Sarkar, M., Madabhavi, I., Niranjan, N., and Dogra, M. (2015). Auscultation of the respiratory system. *Annals of Thoracic Medicine* 10 (3): 158–168.

28 Peak expiratory flow rate

Figure 28.1 Peak expiratory flow rate (PEFR) chart – normal values.
Source: Adapted from Clement Clarke for use with EN13826 / EU scale
peak flow meters from Nunn AJ Gregg I, Br Med J 1989:298; 1068–70.

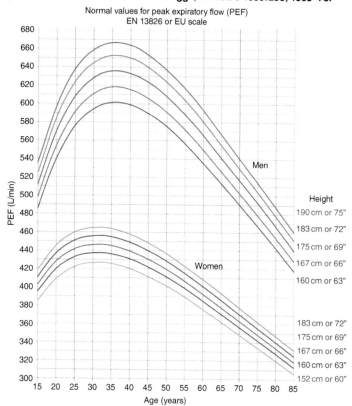

Normal values for peak expiratory flow (PEF)
EN 13826 or EU scale

PEF (L/min) vs Age (years)

Men

Height
190 cm or 75"
183 cm or 72"
175 cm or 69"
167 cm or 66"
160 cm or 63"

Women

183 cm or 72"
175 cm or 69"
167 cm or 66"
160 cm or 63"
152 cm or 60"

Figure 28.3 Correct positioning for obtaining peak expiratory flow rate (PEFR).

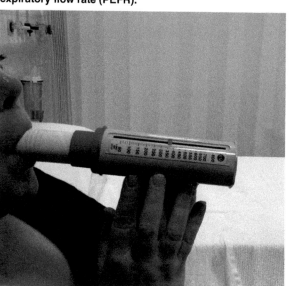

Figure 28.2 Peak flow equipment.

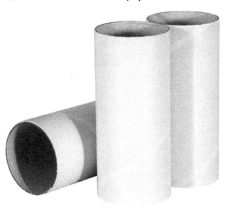

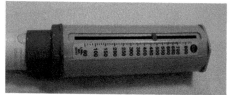

Clinical Nursing Skills at a Glance, First Edition. Edited by Sarah Curr and Carol Fordham-Clarke.
© 2022 John Wiley & Sons Ltd. Published 2022 by John Wiley & Sons Ltd.
Companion website: www.wiley.com/go/clinicalnursingskills

Background

Peak expiratory flow rate (PEFR) measures the maximum rate at which air can be expelled from the lungs through an open mouth. It is a common and simple test of lung function. The PEFR is useful during respiratory assessment as it is a straightforward, quick, assessment method that gives an indication of restriction within the airway. As such it is helpful in assessment and management of patients with asthma as well as patients with other respiratory disorders such as chronic obstructive pulmonary disease (COPD).

The PEFR will often be performed:

- To monitor responses to medication (nebuliser/inhaler) in patients with asthma and COPD.
- To assess the severity of an asthma attack or an exacerbation of COPD.
- To diagnose and monitor patients with asthma.
- PEFR may be required immediately before and 30 minutes after nebulisation to allow for monitoring of the patient's condition.
- Timing of PEFR – this will depend on why PEFR is being measured (Myatt 2017).

NB: Best flow rate should be updated every few years in adults and more frequently in growing children (SIGN and BTS 2019)

Influencing Factors

- As PEFR varies with age, sex, and height, assessment of reduced PEFR should be against a recognised chart of the normal values (Figure 28.1).
- A full A–E assessment, including a respiratory assessment, should be performed prior to obtaining a PEFR, as this is not an appropriate assessment in the acutely unwell adult.
- PEFR is lower in the supine or prone position, so seated or standing should be encouraged (Artunes et al. 2016).

Professional Approach

- Introduce yourself to the patient.
- Fully explain the procedure to obtain informed consent.
- Inform the patient of the results and what they mean if competent to do so.
- Administer any treatments/medication as prescribed.
- Ensure results of the PEFR and any treatment are documented.

Equipment

- Peak expiratory flow rate meter.
- Disposable mouthpiece (Figure 28.2).

Procedure

- Ensure that the patient is standing or sitting as upright as possible to maximise lung expansion.
- Ensure that the position is documented so that the same position can be used for monitoring PEFR.
- Attach the disposable mouthpiece to the peak flow monitor.
- Ensure that the pointer is set to zero.
- Ask the patient to hold the PEFR monitor horizontally.
- Ensure that the fingers are not touching the pointers.
- Ask the patient to take a deep breath in and place lips and teeth around the mouthpiece. Ensure that a tight seal is obtained (Figure 28.3). This may be by asking the patient to place their teeth around the mouthpiece and then close their mouth (Myatt 2017).
- Ask the patient to exhale forcibly as quickly as possible.
- Make a note of the position of the pointer.
- Repeat procedure twice (or, if positioning is poor, up to five times) more. Note the readings.
- Record the highest of the three readings.
- Ensure the patient is comfortable, and inform them of the result.
- Inform a senior nurse and appropriate member of the medical team if the result if abnormal.

Red Flags

- Signs of full or partial respiratory obstruction (i.e. stridor, wheezing) are considered an emergency and PEFR should be stopped immediately and care escalated.
- If there are any signs of respiratory distress (i.e. tachypnoea, central cyanosis), PEFR measurement should not be taken and critical care provided.

References

Artunes, B.O., Dutra de Souza, H.C., Gianinis, H.H. et al. (2016). Peak expiratory flow rate in healthy, young, non-active subjects in seated, supine, and prone postures. *Physiotherapy Theory and Practice*. 32 (6): 489–493.

Myatt, R. (2017). Measuring peak expiratory flow rate: what the nurse needs to know. *Nursing Standard* 32 (20): 40–44.

Scottish Intercollegiate Guidelines Network (SIGN) & British Thoracic Society (BTS) (2019). *SIGN 158: British Guideline on the Management of Asthma*. https://www.sign.ac.uk/media/1773/sign158-updated.pdf (accessed 20 May 2021).

29 Administering oxygen

Figure 29.1   Nasal cannulae.

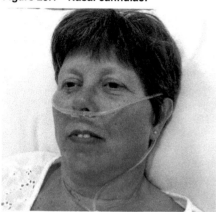

Table 29.1 Safety considerations.

Oxygen is highly inflammable and supports combustion and thus an awareness of safety is essential:
* Oxygen cylinders should be kept secure, in an upright position and away from heat
* Smoking is prohibited in the vicinity of oxygen
* Naked flames are prohibited in the vicinity of oxygen
* Care is required if high-flow oxygen is in use when using a defibrillator
* Alcohol, ether, and inflammatory liquids must be used with caution around oxygen

Figure 29.2   Venturi and mask.

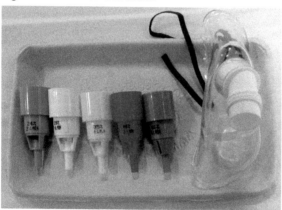

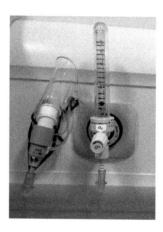

Figure 29.3   Non-rebreathe mask.

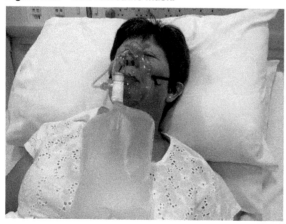

Figure 29.4   Comfortable and secure oxygen devices.

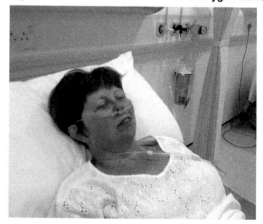

Clinical Nursing Skills at a Glance, First Edition. Edited by Sarah Curr and Carol Fordham-Clarke.
© 2022 John Wiley & Sons Ltd. Published 2022 by John Wiley & Sons Ltd.
Companion website: www.wiley.com/go/clinicalnursingskills

Background

Oxygen can be described as a colourless, odourless, tasteless, and transparent gas. This gas is contained within the air we breathe and is essential for life. One of the principal functions of the human respiratory system is to deliver this oxygen to the tissues while also removing metabolic waste products. If this respiratory system is impaired, additional oxygen administration may well be required. In emergency situations high-flow oxygen (15 L via a non-rebreathe mask) can be administered (O'Driscoll et al. 2017) without a prescription but in most instances the person will need to be reviewed before oxygen is prescribed.

Influencing Factors – Indications for Oxygen Therapy

- *Type 1 respiratory failure*. This in when the patient has a low oxygen level (hypoxaemic) and the carbon dioxide level is normal. This is commonly seen in patients with pulmonary oedema, pneumonia, and infective conditions of the lungs.
- *Type 2 respiratory failure*. The patient has a low oxygen level with a raised carbon dioxide level. This is referred to as hypercapnia and is commonly seen in patients with chronic obstructive pulmonary disorder (COPD), in respiratory muscle weakness as well as in chest injury.
- In the critically unwell patient, high-flow oxygen is often indicated (NICE 2007), i.e. in severe asthma, sepsis, hypovolaemia, or acute myocardial infarction.
- During anaesthesia.
- Post-operatively.

Professional Approach

- Introduce yourself to the patient.
- Explain procedure and obtain informed consent.
- Document the results of all treatments.
- Ensure that the nurse in charge/appropriate member of the medical team is informed of any changes in the patient's condition.

Equipment

Different devices will be used depending on the reason for oxygen administration, including:

- Nasal cannula (Figure 29.1).
- Simple oxygen mask.
- Oxygen mask and Venturi (Figure 29.2).
- Non-rebreathe oxygen mask (Figure 29.3).

Procedure

- Ensure oxygen is prescribed (unless it is an emergency).
- Select an appropriate device for administering oxygen.
- Consider the need for humidification.
- Assemble all the required equipment.
- Explain the procedure to the patient.
- Decontaminate hands.
- Turn the oxygen on to the required flow rate.

   NB: Usually the centre of the ball in the flow meter must sit at the level of the flow rate prescribed but manufacturer's instructions should always be checked.

- Place the mask over the patient's face/nasal cannulae into the nostrils.
- Ensure the oxygen-delivering device is fixed comfortably and securely (Figure 29.4).
- Monitor the oxygen saturations and measure the respiratory rate (Chapter 25). It is also imperative to observe the patient for signs of distress as well as compliance and to ensure that they are comfortable.
- Document/sign prescription as appropriate.

   Safety considerations are outlined in Table 29.1.

Humidification

This will be required if the person is receiving high-flow oxygen for more than 24 hours or is experiencing discomfort as a result of dryness (O'Driscoll et al. 2017). It should also be considered:

- If the patient has thick secretions and is having trouble coughing them up (expectorating).
- If the patient has a tracheostomy.

Red Flags

- Oxygen therapy must be prescribed except in emergency situations.
- Oxygen should be used cautiously in patients who are hypercapnic and retain carbon dioxide due to COPD. Oxygen is usually only administered at 24–28% and the patient should be carefully monitored in case of adverse effects.

References

National Institute of Health and Care Excellence (2007). *CG50 Acutely Ill Adults in Hospital: Recognising and Responding to Deterioration*. London: National Institute of Health and Care Excellence.

O'Driscoll, B.R., Howard, L., Earis, J. et al. (2017). BTS guideline for oxygen for oxygen use in adults in healthcare and emergency settings. *Thorax* 72 (1): i1–i88.

30 Nebulisers and inhalers

Figure 30.1 Spacer with mouthpiece (a) and mask (b).

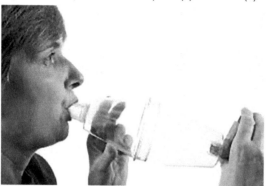

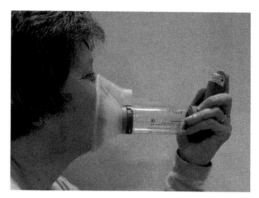

Figure 30.2 Nebuliser (a) and equipment (b).

Figure 30.3 Nebuliser with mouthpiece.

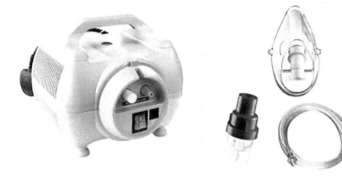

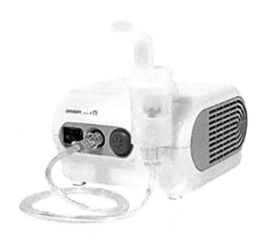

Background

Inhalers provide medication into the lungs with minimal side-effects (Scullion 2020) and are thus quicker-acting and more effective than their oral counterparts. These medications can be bronchodilators, often used for chronic obstructive pulmonary disorder (COPD) and asthma exacerbation, or corticosteroids for longer-term management which prevent the inflammatory process from initiating. These inhalers come in three different categories:

- Metered dose.
- Breathe-actuated.
- Dry power (BMA and RPS 2020).

As it has been suggested that as many as 86% of people using an inhaler have a poor technique (Lavorini et al. 2020) it is recommended that spacers are used with a metered dose inhaler (Figure 30.1) to ensure effective administration (Shealy et al. 2017).

If respiratory needs are not met, then a nebuliser may well be required. With jet nebulisation the compressed air or gas breaks the nebulised solution into smaller particles, resulting in the solution forming a fine mist (Bardsley et al. 2018) which is inhaled via a face mask or mouthpiece (Figures 30.2 and 30.3).

Influencing Factors

To ensure that the patient can self-administer effectively, both knowledge of technique and dexterity to perform need to be considered (Booth 2020). As such, conditions that affect dexterity need to be considered, as do conditions that affect cognition and knowledge retention. The healthcare professional must take a full history to ensure that the most appropriate medication is prescribed.

As nebulised medication can be administered with compressed gas or air, the patient's holistic needs must be considered. As there has been suggestion that compressed air is more beneficial than oxygen for exacerbation of COPD (Bardsley et al. 2018), the prescriber needs to consider which adjunct to use. Both need to be administered at a flow rate of 6 L/minute (O'Driscoll et al. 2017).

Professional Approach

- Explain the procedure to obtain informed consent.
- Ensure that you are aware of the action of different inhalers to enable you to teach the patient how to use it correctly.
- Ensure that the required medication checks are followed throughout the procedure.

Equipment – Inhaler

- Appropriate inhaler.
- Spacer as required.

Equipment – Nebulisation

- Jet or ultrasonic nebuliser set.
- Face mask or another appropriate device.
- Connection tubing.

Procedure – Administering a nebuliser

- Follow the nine rights of medication administration (Elliot and Liu 2010).
- Explain the required steps to the patient.
- Prepare the device or prepare and load dose.
- Ask the patient to breathe out.
- Place the inhaler into the spacer as per manufacturer's instructions as required.
- Place mouth around the mouthpiece, forming a seal with the lips.

- For metered dose and breath, actuated inhalers breathe in and out slowly at a consistent pace.
- For dry powder inhalers, breathe in quickly and deeply.
- Hold breath for 10 seconds if not using a spacer.
- Repeat as required.

NB: If using a spacer, it should be washed once a week in accordance with manufacturer's guidance.

Procedure – Administering a Nebuliser

- Assemble all equipment.
- Follow the nine rights of medication and ensure that a compressed gas has been prescribed.
- Encourage the patient to sit up.
- Place the liquid medication into the nebuliser chamber.
- Attach to the tubing.
- Attach the tubing to the mouthpiece/face mask, ensuring that it is correctly sized, well fitted, and comfortable.
- Set the flow rate to 6 L/minute (O'Driscoll et al. 2017).
- Ensure that a fine mist is seen and that a hissing sound is heard.
- Follow the guidance of medication manufacturers regarding administration time period, usually 10–15 minutes.
- Nebulisers may cause the patient to cough, so ensure that tissues and a sputum pot are readily available.
- Document on the electronic or paper medication administration record that the drug has been delivered.

NB: A peak flow may be required before nebulised solution and 20 minutes after the drug has been administered. Information on how to perform this can be found in Chapter 28.

Red Flags

- Patients using nebulisers must be observed for toleration and signs of respiratory distress.
- Teaching the patient to use the inhaler correctly is critical to ensure the delivery of the medication.
- A silent chest is a clinical emergency and will most likely require intubation.

References

Bardsley, G., Pilcher, J., McKinstry, S., Shirtcliffe, P., Weatherall, M. & Beasley, R. (2018) Oxygen versus air-driven nebulisers for exacerbations of chronic obstructive pulmonary disease: a randomised controlled trial. *BMC Pulmonary Medicine* 18: 157. https://www.ncbi.nlm.nih.gov/pmc/articles/PMC6171193 (accessed 21 July /2020).

Booth, A. (2020). Inhaled therapy for asthma. *Practice Nursing* 2 (6): 300–309.

British Medical Association & Royal Pharmaceutical Press (2020). *British National Formulary (BNF) 79*. London: Pharmaceutical Press.

Elliot, M. and Liu, Y. (2010). The *nine rights* of medication administration: an overview. *British Journal of Nursing* 19 (5): 300–305.

Lavorini, F., Barreto, C., van Boven, J.F.M. et al. (2020). Spacer & Valved Holding Chambers – the risk of switching to different chambers. *Journal of Allergy and Clinical Immunology: In Practice* 8 (5): 1569–1573.

O'Driscoll, B.R., Howard, L., Earis, J. et al. (2017). BTS guideline for oxygen for oxygen use in adults in healthcare and emergency settings. *Thorax* 72 (1): i1–i188.

Scullion, J. (2020). Teaching inhaler technique. *Journal of Prescribing Practice* 2 (5): 234–237.

Shealy, K.M., Pardiso, V.C., Slimmer, M.L. et al. (2017). Evaluation of the prevalence and effectiveness of education on metered dose inhaler technique. *Respiratory Care* 62 (7): 882–887. Publication Type Language.

31 Tracheostomy care

Figure 31.1 Tracheostomy tubes.

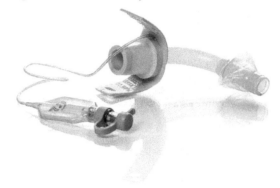

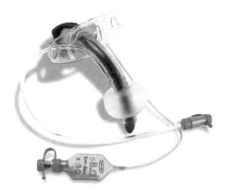

Figure 31.2 Tracheostomy safety equipment.

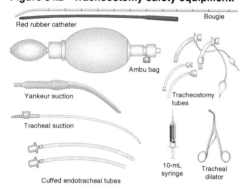

Red rubber catheter
Bougie
Ambu bag
Yankeur suction
Tracheostomy tubes
Tracheal suction
Cuffed endotracheal tubes
10-mL syringe
Tracheal dilator

Figure 31.3 Heat moisture exchange.

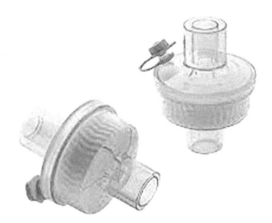

Figure 31.4 Tracheostomy dressing change.

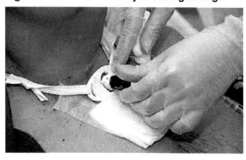

Table 31.1 Types of tracheostomy tube.

Type	Description
Cuffed tubes	Tube with inflatable cuff. The cuff creates a seal that prevents aspiration. Also if the patient is ventilated it stops air from leaking around the tracheostomy **NB:** Although the cuff is inflated the patient will not be able to talk as no air is moving across the vocal cords Most commonly seen/ used
Uncuffed tubes	Not as common as cuffed tubes but used in patients who can breathe unaided and who have a normal swallow reflex
Fenestrated tubes	Fenestrations or holes are situated on the upper side of the tube. There is matching inner tube with holes and one without holes. These tubes allow air/secretions to pass into the oral and nasal cavity. This allows patients to get used to breathing naturally again

Clinical Nursing Skills at a Glance, First Edition. Edited by Sarah Curr and Carol Fordham-Clarke.
© 2022 John Wiley & Sons Ltd. Published 2022 by John Wiley & Sons Ltd.
Companion website: www.wiley.com/go/clinicalnursingskills

Background

A tracheostomy is an opening (stoma) into the trachea. This opening is performed surgically (by a surgeon in the operating theatre) or percutaneously (in the intensive care unit). A tube is then inserted into the hole. This allows for breathing and the removal of secretions and can be temporary or more permanent. As such, care and safety checks will need to be provided.

Influencing Factors – Indications for a Tracheostomy

- To provide a secure, patent airway to support and maintain respirations.
- As an aid to weaning patients from ventilatory support in the intensive care setting.
- If the patient has required major head or neck surgery.
- If the patient has had a major head or neck trauma.
- To enable the effective removal of secretions from the respiratory tract.
- If the patient has vocal cord paralysis.
- If there is an impaired swallow reflex and the patient is likely to aspirate.

Influencing Factors – Complications Associated with Tracheostomies

- Infection.
- Bleeding.
- Blockage.
- Thickening of the tracheal wall resulting in tracheal stenosis.
- Displacement or accidental removal of the tracheostomy.
- Ulceration.

Professional Approach

- Always introduce yourself to the patient.
- Provide explanations, ensure that the patient can communicate, and document all actions clearly.
- Ensure you are fully aware of how to care for a patient with a tracheostomy.
- Ensure you are familiar with all the emergency procedures required for a patient with a tracheostomy.
- Become familiar with local policy/tracheostomy care bundles.
- Providing support for the patient and family members is essential, particularly for those with a new tracheostomy, where there will be adjustments and changes in body image.

Equipment – Tracheostomy Tubes

The normal adult tracheostomy tube size is 7.0–8.5 mm internal diameter (Figure 31.1). Although there are several different types of tube (Table 31.1), most will have an inner tube which will reduce the inner diameter slightly. The inner tube should be changed regularly (according to local guidance) in order to prevent secretion building up on the inner wall of the tube. The tube size must also be documented in the patient's notes and checked daily.

- Safety equipment – always kept by the patient (Figure 31.2).
- Spare tracheostomy tubes (same size and smaller).
- Spare inner tube and tracheal dilators (in case of tracheostomy dislodgement).
- Humidification – all tracheostomies require humidification (heated or cold-water systems). Alternatively heat moisture exchangers can be used as they reflect warmth and moisture back into the airways (Figure 31.3).

Procedure – Tracheostomy Care

The National Tracheostomy Safety Project (NTSP) provides a checklist of daily activities which include:

- Assessing the stoma site daily and checking for signs of infection (NTSP 2013a); cleaning the site with 0.9% sodium chloride as required.
- Checking the dressing daily and changing when soiled using aseptic non-touch technique. The tracheostomy tapes hold the tube in position and thus require two healthcare professionals to change them. One holds the tube in position, preventing displacement, and the other ties the tapes (Figure 31.4).
- Daily checks of the secure device holding the tracheostomy (Everitt 2016) to assess for signs of dislodgment and pressure ulcers.
- Checking the internal cannula for secretion build-up.

Procedure – Communication

Patients are unable to verbalise as there is no air passing over their vocal cords. Provide pens/ paper, writing boards, signs and alphabet boards. Liaise with occupational therapy to help with communication aids. The call bell must be left nearby at all times.

Procedure – Nutrition

- Swallowing can be difficult/impaired with a tracheostomy tube. Prior to commencement of oral fluids and food, the patient must have a swallow assessment by the speech and language therapists.
- Dieticians should be involved to ensure that the patient has adequate nutrition. If they are unable to swallow, consider nasogastric feeding (Chapter 41).

Procedure – Suctioning

- Routine clearing of secretions from the respiratory tract using suction will be required and it is suggested that this is completed every eight hours and should be limited to the lumen of the tube (NTSP 2013b).
- Secretions can be removed from the oral cavity only using a Yankauer sucker.
- Deep tracheal suctioning requires additional training to achieve competence and ensure patient safety. It is important that the appropriate catheter size is chosen and that the required suction pressure is maintained.
- Prior to considering suctioning, the competent individual should encourage the person to cough and support them into a position for this (NTSP 2013b). Regular chest physiotherapy will also be required.

Red Flags

- A blocked or displaced tracheostomy tube is a medical emergency and requires immediate action.
- If suctioning, you must ensure you receive appropriate training and maintain competence, as trachea damage and hypoxia can occur with an improperly sized suction catheter and excessive pressure.

References

Everitt, K. (2016). Caring for patients with a tracheostomy. *Nursing Times* 112 (19): 16–20.

National Tracheostomy Safety Project (2013a) *Daily Checks*. www.tracheostomy.org.uk/storage/files/Daily%20checks.pdf (accessed 31 October 2020).

National Tracheostomy Safety Project (2013b) *Suctioning*. www.tracheostomy.org.uk/storage/files/Suctioning.pdf (accessed 31 October 2020).

32 Chest drain management

Figure 32.1 Chest drain insertion site. *Source*: Redrawn from Davey (2014).

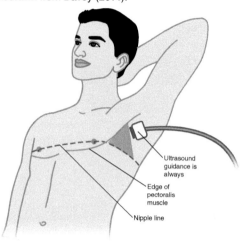

Ultrasound guidance is always

Edge of pectoralis muscle

Nipple line

Figure 32.2 Chest drains.

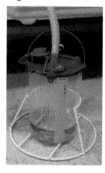
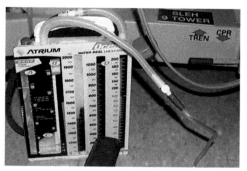

Figure 32.3 Chest drain dressing.

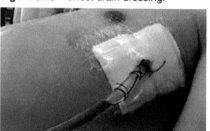
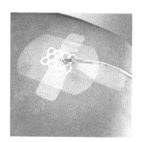

Table 32.1 Mechanisms of a chest drain.

A clear plastic thoracostomy tube of appropriate diameter
A draining unit bottle
A one-way mechanism, provided by a water seal or valve
The proximal end of the drainage tube is inserted into the pleura and the distal end is connected to the drainage system. During exhalation, positive pressure in the thorax forces air and liquid out of the pleural cavity and into the drainage system until normal negative intrapleural pressure returns
A one-bottle system is the most common (Figure 32.2a) – but increasingly plastic multi-chamber units are being used (Figure 32.2b) (George and Papagiannopoulos 2016) – follow manufacturer's instructions
Continuous low negative pressure (–5 kPa) suction may be applied to the drainage unit where there is a persistent air leak or large fluid collection to further promote drainage and extraction of air

Table 32.2 Indications for chest drainage

A chest drain will often be inserted when a patient presents with:
- Tension pneumothorax
- Bilateral pneumothorax
- Large pleural effusion
- Spontaneous pneumothorax
- Traumatic haemothorax
- Chylothorax
- Post-surgical – thoracotomy, oesophagectomy, cardiothoracic surgery
- Empyema.

Table 32.3 Indications for clamping a chest drain.

- Following rapid initial drainage (>1500 mL in the first hour)
- During collection unit or bottle change
- Disconnection of the drainage tube from the collection bottle
- Following drug instillation into the drainage tube, for a brief period as per medical instruction

Source: Adapted from Woodrow (2013).

Table 32.4 Troubleshooting possible problems.

Loss of drainage	Remove any kinks from the tubing and ensure the container is below the chest. Change tubing if it is blocked
Drainage tubing is disconnected from the drain	Clamp tube immediately. Reconnect as soon as possible, using a clean, sterile system if possible, and unclamp. Notify medical staff of incident
Collecting container falls over	Stand bottle upright again immediately and observe the patient. Inform medical staff
Chest tube falls out	Tie the purse-string suture immediately. Inform medical staff and conduct a patient assessment, including full vital signs

Clinical Nursing Skills at a Glance, First Edition. Edited by Sarah Curr and Carol Fordham-Clarke.
© 2022 John Wiley & Sons Ltd. Published 2022 by John Wiley & Sons Ltd.
Companion website: www.wiley.com/go/clinicalnursingskills

Background

An intrapleural chest drain is a tube inserted into the space between the parietal and visceral pleura which surround the lungs (Figure 32.1). This pleural cavity is usually filled with 5–15 mL of fluid (Kiefer 2017), which allows the pleural layers to slide against each other during inspiration and exhalation. The aim of the chest drain is to drain accumulations of fluid or air from the pleural space (Woodrow 2013). This prevents collapse and compression of the lung and enables re-expansion. Details of how a chest drain works can be found in Table 32.1.

Influencing Factors

Refer to indications for chest drainage, Table 32.2

Professional Approach

- A patient with an intrapleural drain should be nursed by someone competent in the care and management of the drain and the possible complications.
- The healthcare professional must provide education for ongoing care to the client and their family or carers.

Procedure – Chest Drain Management

After chest drain insertion:

- Ensure that a chest X-ray is taken immediately after insertion to assess position and note any complications.
- Ensure a transparent dressing (Figure 32.3) has been applied, for visibility of insertion site. Monitor daily for signs of infection and discharge, change as indicated.
- Attach the drainage bottle to an underwater seal, ensuring the tube in the collecting bottle is under 2 cm of water (Figure 32.2).
- Observe for movement of the water column in the drainage bottle or tubing:
  - spontaneous bubbling due to pneumothorax.
  - "swinging" in time with respirations once air is removed.
- Observe drain fluid output, noting colour and consistency, mark the level on the bottle, and document on the fluid chart.
- Observe drain output and bubbling initially half-hourly then every one to four hours depending on patient condition and fluid loss.
- Report sudden increases in drainage of > 100 mL/hour to the relevant medical team.
- Where possible, nurse the patient sitting up at 45° with regular observation of vital signs and respiratory assessment. Encourage deep breaths and mobilise as permitted.
- Administer regular pain relief as required.
- Report any breathlessness, coughing, or chest pain immediately.
- Ensure the bottle remains below waist height to prevent backflow of drain contents into the pleural space and is secured in a stand (Figure 32.2a) or to the bed to prevent accidental falling over.
- Observe for kinks in the tubing or obstructions that could impede drainage.
- Only clamp the drain when changing the bottle or after accidental disconnection, unclamping as soon as possible (Table 32.3) to minimise the risk of developing a tension pneumothorax.
- Change the drainage unit after 500 mL of drainage or every three days using an aseptic technique.

- Awareness of drainage problems is essential as these may influence the patient's respiratory function (Millar and Hillman, 2018). Refer to Table 32.4.

Equipment – Chest Drain Removal

- Non-sterile gloves and disposable apron.
- Wound care pack with sterile gloves in correct size.
- Stitch cutter.
- Sterile, transparent dressing.

Procedure – Chest Drain Removal

- Chest drain removal follows medical instruction, cessation of air leak and fluid drainage, and a satisfactory chest X-ray.
- Removal requires two nurses competent in the technique – one to pull out the drain and one to tie the mattress suture, wearing personal protective equipment, including goggles or visor (Allibone 2015).
- Administer pain relief allowing time for effect.
- Sit the patient up, obtain informed consent, and discuss the breathing technique that the patient should take, if able; allow time for practise of these techniques.
- Prior to the procedure, inspect the mattress suture to ensure it will close the site once pulled. Request a further suture if necessary.
- Decontaminate hands.
- Prepare wound dressing pack.
- Apply disposable apron and sterile gloves.
- Cut the suture anchoring the drain to the skin.
- Instruct the patient to take three deep breathes and then hold their breath (bearing down if possible, in a Valsalva manoeuvre). This minimises the risk of introducing air into the pleura via the drain site.
- Ensure one nurse pulls out the drain quickly and smoothly, and immediately on removal ensure that the other nurse quickly ties the mattress suture to close the incision.
- Cover with a transparent dressing.
- Ensure a repeat chest X-ray occurs after drain removal.
- Document actions as well as rationale for removal.
- Remove the mattress suture 7–10 days later as per local policy.

Red Flags

- Never clamp a bubbling chest drain, as it could result in a tension pneumothorax.
- Chest drains should not be "milked" using roller clamps as this generates high negative pleural pressures.
- Observe the subcutaneous tissue around the insertion site for air infiltration (surgical emphysema) which may compromise the patient's air entry. This can occur if a drainage hole is positioned outside the pleural cavity or if tubing is blocked or kinked.

References

Allibone, E. (2015). How to remove a chest drain. *Nursing Standard* 30 (6): 34–36.

George, G.S. and Papagiannopoulos, K. (2016). Advances in chest drain management in thoracic disease. *Journal of Thoracic Disease* 8 (Suppl 1): S55–S64.

Kiefer, T. (2017). *Chest Drains in Daily Clinical Practice*. Cham, Springer Nature.

Millar, F.R. and Hillman, T. (2018). Managing chest drains on medical wards. *British Medical Journal* 363 (k4639): 1–7.

Woodrow, P. (2013). Intrapleural chest drainage. *Nursing Standard* 27 (40): 49–56.

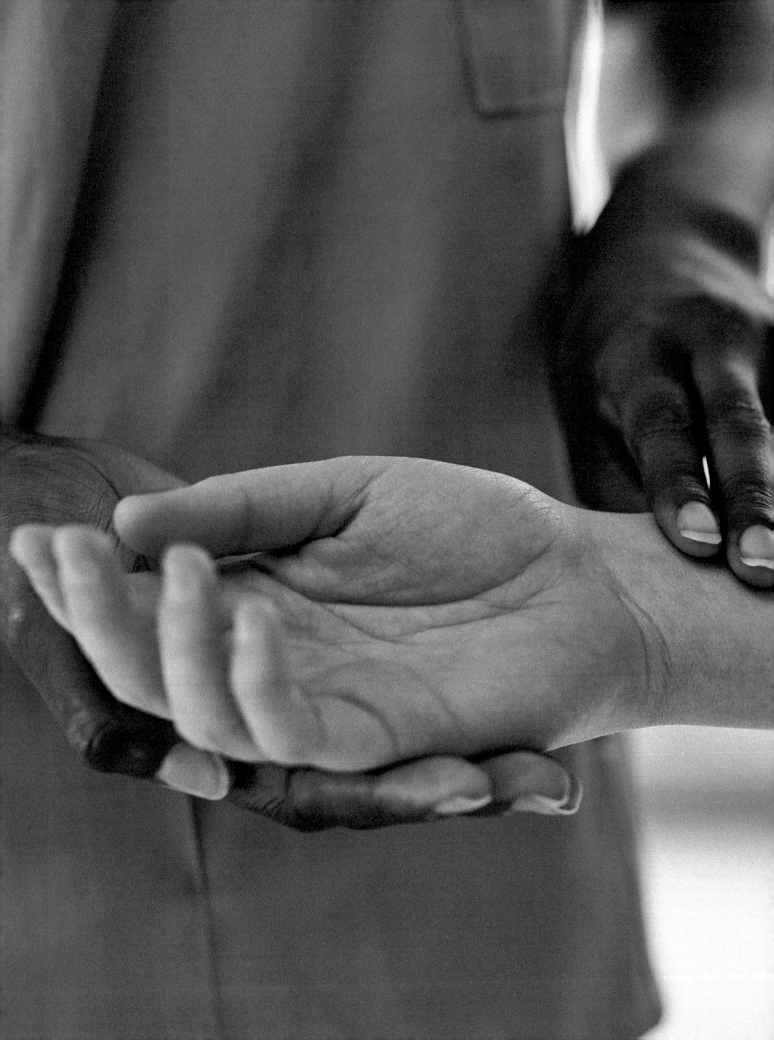

Cardiovascular skills

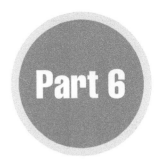

Part 6

Chapters

33 Taking a pulse

Figure 33.1   Pulse sites.

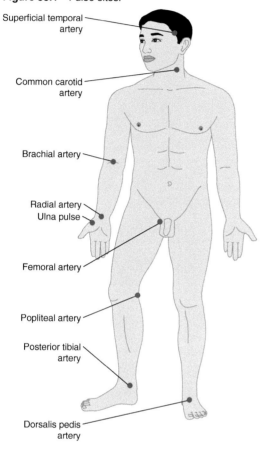

Superficial temporal artery
Common carotid artery
Brachial artery
Radial artery
Ulna pulse
Femoral artery
Popliteal artery
Posterior tibial artery
Dorsalis pedis artery

Figure 33.2   Taking a radial pulse.

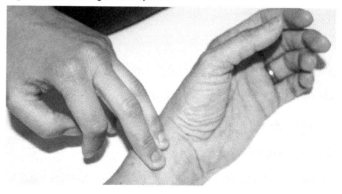

Figure 33.3   Documenting a pulse.

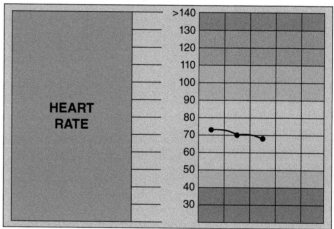

HEART RATE

>140
130
120
110
100
90
80
70
60
50
40
30

Table 33.1 Interpreting the pulse.

Normal range	60–90 beats/minute in a resting adult
Tachycardia	Pulse rate > 90 beats/minute
Bradycardia	Pulse rate < 60 beats/minute

Table 33.2 Assessing the quality of the pulse (pulse score).

0	Pulse absent
1+	Pulse difficult to palpate, weak, thready, easily obliterated
2+	Normal pulse, easily palpated, not easily obliterated
3+	Strong, bounding, easily palpated, cannot be obliterated

Clinical Nursing Skills at a Glance, First Edition. Edited by Sarah Curr and Carol Fordham-Clarke.
© 2022 John Wiley & Sons Ltd. Published 2022 by John Wiley & Sons Ltd.
Companion website: www.wiley.com/go/clinicalnursingskills

Background

The cardiac cycle comprises systole (contraction) and diastole (relaxation). Blood is ejected from the heart into arterial circulation during the systole part of this cycle. The arteries expand as they receive the blood pumped from the heart and contract with elastic recoil during diastole. This rhythmic pressure wave is carried along the arteries and can be manually palpated as a pulse. A pulse can be felt where the arteries lie close to the body surface or over a bony prominence. It is this pulse rate that represents the heart rate, one of the five vital signs.

The rate at which the heart pumps can be affected by a number of factors (see "Influencing factors") and it is necessary to be aware of these factors prior to undertaking this skill. Equally, the rhythm of the heart can be affected by underlying medical conditions, medications, and electrolyte imbalances. Although a normal pulse rate is regular, if there are problems with the conduction system in the heart, an irregular rhythm can occur (Calkins et al. 2012). The most common defect in conduction is atrial fibrillation (NICE 2014), which is when conduction in the atrium is chaotic and these additional impulses affect the normal conduction that starts from the sino-atrial node.

The amplitude/volume of the pulse is affected by the strength of contraction and elasticity of the artery wall, but it can be also affected by any disorder that impacts on haemodynamic circulation and thus cardiac output.

Pulse Sites

- The radial pulses are easily accessed and are those most commonly used.
- Central pulses such as the carotids and femorals are useful in situations where there is circulatory insufficiency or where peripheral pulses may be absent or difficult to palpate.
- Lower limb pulses are important when assessing for compromised regional blood flow.
- Familiarise yourself with all pulse sites and use the most appropriate site for your assessment (Figure 33.1).

Influencing Factors

The heart rate relies on a balance between the parasympathetic and sympathetic nervous system and should usually be between 60 and 90 beats/minute (**bpm**) at rest (Waugh and Grant 2018). There are numerous factors that can affect the heart rate, the most common of which are:

- Exercise.
- Sleep.
- Emotion.
- Hormonal fluctuations.
- Temperature.
- Anger/excitement/fear.
- Medication – illegal and legal.
- Caffeine.
- Nicotine.
- Alcohol.

Professional Approach

- Explain the procedure and ensure that it is understood to obtain informed consent.
- Use the most readily available pulse, usually the radial, and re-obtain consent if you need to move to another site.
- Be mindful that the sense of privacy and dignity will differ between individuals and provide privacy when asked or when exposing a site that is not socially exposed.

Equipment

- Alcohol hand rub.
- Watch with a second hand.

Procedure

- Ensure the patient is comfortable and relaxed.
- Establish if there are any factors that could affect the reading.
- Select the appropriate site for taking the pulse and obtain informed consent.
- Place two fingers on the pulse site (Figure 33.2) (the first and second or second and third fingers can be used – the thumb has a strong pulse so should not be used).
- Apply gentle pressure and maintain this while you count the rate for 60 seconds. Counting for less and multiplying to get bpm can lead to inaccuracies.
- Document on the appropriate chart (Figure 33.3).
- Note any irregularities in the rate (Table 33.1), the rhythm,[1] and amplitude (Table 33.2).
- Document the pulse in bpm as per local guidance.

Interpreting a Pulse

- A normal pulse is regular and easily palpated.
- Pulse quality is indicative of circulating blood volume.
- Abnormal findings should be reported to the nurse in charge and an appropriate member of the medical team.

Red Flags

- Absent pulse
- Weak thready pulse
- An irregular pulse must be counted for 60 seconds.

References

Calkins, H., Kuck, K.H., Cappato, R. et al. (2012). HRS/EHRA/ECAS expert consensus statement on catheter and surgical ablation of atrial fibrillation: recommendations for patient selection, procedural techniques, patient management and follow-up, definitions, endpoints, and research trial design. *Journal of Interventional Cardiac Electrophysiology* 33 (2): 171–257.

NICE (2014) *Atrial Fibrillation: Management. Clinical Guideline [CG180].* www.nice.org.uk/guidance/cg180/resources/atrial-fibrillation-management-pdf-35109805981381 (accessed 20 May 2021).

Waugh, A. and Grant, A. (2018). *Ross & Wilson Anatomy and Physiology: In Health and Illness*, 13e. London: Elsevier.

1 The pulse can be regular (normal) or irregular. If the pulse is irregular document if it is irregularly irregular or regularly irregular. This will give insight into the underlying cause.

34 Blood pressure

Figure 34.1 Manual blood pressure equipment.

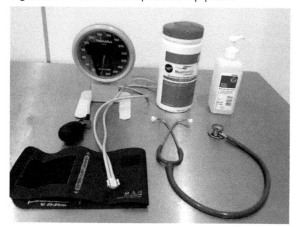

Figure 34.2 Choosing the correct cuff.

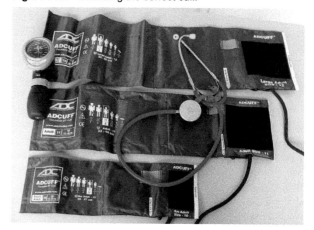

Figure 34.3 Correct cuff and stethoscope position.

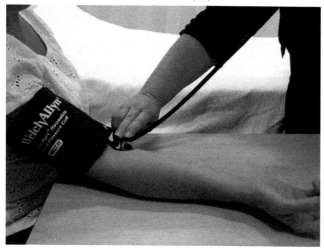

Figure 34.4 Documenting blood pressure.

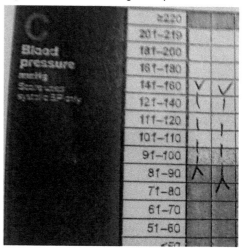

Clinical Nursing Skills at a Glance, First Edition. Edited by Sarah Curr and Carol Fordham-Clarke.
© 2022 John Wiley & Sons Ltd. Published 2022 by John Wiley & Sons Ltd.
Companion website: www.wiley.com/go/clinicalnursingskills

Background

In order to maintain adequate circulation, the heart needs to pump effectively and pump enough blood around the body. It is this pumping of the heart and the pressure gradient generated between the arterial and venous circulations that maintains blood flow around the body.

Blood pressure (BP) is the pressure in the arteries during the phases of the cardiac cycle and can be defined as the force exerted by the blood on the walls of the arteries.

Blood pressure considers two pressures in the arteries: the systolic pressure, which is the pressure created during cardiac contraction; and diastolic pressure, which is the pressure when the heart rests between beats.

- Systolic pressure is determined by the cardiac output (CO).
- CO is determined by the stroke volume (SV), the amount of blood ejected by the left ventricle in one contraction, multiplied by the heart rate (HR), the number of beats felt in one minute (CO= SV × HR).
- Diastolic pressure is the amount of resistance to blood flow, the systemic vascular resistance (SVR) This is the combined resistance of all the blood vessels, but in humans it is predominantly determined by the diameter of the arterioles.
- An average BP or mean arterial pressure (MABP) can be expressed as:

$$MABP = CO \times SVR$$

Influencing Factors

- White coat effect.
- Exercise.
- Stress and anxiety.
- Drugs/medications/caffeine.
- Inaccurate procedures[1].

Equipment (Figure 34.1)

- Sphygmomanometer.
- Appropriately sized cuff – the bladder within the cuff should cover 80% of the circumference of the upper arm (BIHS 2017) (Figure 34.2).
- Stethoscope for taking a manual BP.

Procedure – Manual BP

- Ensure that all equipment is in good working order and has been calibrated within the previous six months.
- Ensure the sphygmomanometer dial rests at zero.
- Clean the earpieces and stethoscope diaphragm using an alcohol-based solution according to local policy.
- Ensure the patient is in a comfortable position and is relaxed with their arm supported and palm facing upwards.
- Remove any tight or restrictive clothing around the upper arm.
- Place the sphygmomanometer level with the patient's heart.
- Palpate the patient's brachial artery.

---

1 A manual BP should be recorded in pregnancy, after a hypotension or hypertension recording, in trauma, and when an arrythmia is noted.

- Wrap the cuff around the patient's upper arm so that the centre of the bladder covers the brachial artery and the lower edge of the cuff is 2–3 cm above the antecubital fossa (Figure 34.3).
- Ensure the sphygmomanometer dial is level with the patient's heart.
- Estimate the systolic pressure by inflating the cuff until the radial pulse is no longer felt.
- Deflate the cuff completely and make a note of the point at which the pulse disappeared.
- Wait 15–30 seconds before re-inflating the cuff to obtain the BP reading. The cuff will need to be inflated to 30 mmHg above the estimated systolic pressure (BIHS 2017). This is performed to avoid underestimating the systolic pressure due to an auscultatory gap.
- Position the stethoscope over the brachial artery (Figure 34.3).
- Deflate the cuff at a rate of 2 mmHg/second, while listening for Korotkoff sounds (BIHS 2017).
- Five distinct phases of Korotkoff sounds occur as the cuff deflates.
- The first sound, often described as a loud tap or sharp thud, is the systolic pressure reading.
- The diastolic pressure reading is taken when all sounds cease.
- Once the readings have been obtained, fully deflate the cuff, remove, and ensure the patient is made comfortable.
- Clean all equipment.
- Document (Figure 34.4) and report abnormalities. Informing the senior nurse or doctor as required by NEWS.

Procedure – Electronic BP

- Follow individual manufacturers' guidelines.
- Ensure the correct cuff size is used.
- Ensure the machine is reset between patients.
- Ensure infection control procedures are followed.

Professional Approach

- Ensure that informed consent is obtained.
- Consider any contraindications, i.e. exercise, medication.
- Maintain privacy and dignity.

Red Flags

- Hypotension with other cardiovascular signs could be indicative of shock and requires emergency intervention.
- Electronic devices frequently fail to register low BP and arrythmias (NICE 2019). Staff must remain competent to perform a manual BP reading.
- In pregnancy Korotkoff sounds may persist to zero. In this instance the diastolic reading should be taken at the point when muffling of sounds occurs (sound 4).

References

British and Irish Hypertension Society (2017). *Blood Pressure Management: Using Manual Blood Pressure Monitors.* Leicester: British and Irish Hypertension Society.

National Institute for Health and Care Excellence (2019). *NG 136 Hypertension in Adults: Diagnosis and Management.* London: National Institute for Health and Care Excellence.

35 Temperature assessment

Figure 35.1 Oral thermometer placement.

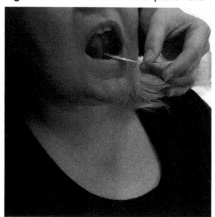

Figure 35.2 Chemical dot reading.

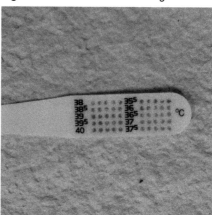

Figure 35.3 Taking the tympanic temperature with ear tug.

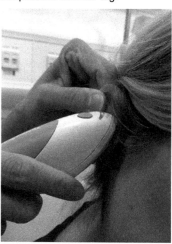

Figure 35.4 Correct documentation.

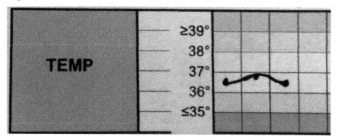

Table 35.1 Thermoregulation.

Mechanisms activated by cold	Mechanisms activated by heat
Heat gain • Shivering – thermogenesis as a result of intense muscular contraction • Activation of sympathetic activity with adrenaline and noradrenaline to increase basal metabolic rate • Activation of thyroid hormones to increase metabolism – hunger	**Heat loss** • Cutaneous vasodilatation – more blood brought to skin surface with increased heat loss via radiation, convection • Sweating – increased heat loss through evaporation • Increased respiration – water loss
Prevention of heat loss • Horripilation – goosebumps reduce heat loss from skin via convection and radiation • Vasocontriction – prevents heat loss from blood at skin surface • Voluntary activity – warm clothing, curling up, hot food and drinks	**Decreased heat production** • Anorexia • Apathy • Cooler clothing, cold drinks

Table 35.2 Abnormal temperature states.

Abnormal temperature states	Definition
Fever	A regulated rise in core temperature. The hypothalamus resets the body's thermostat to a higher setting in response to infection or inflammation. Homeostatic responses are triggered that raise the temperature of the blood. Counter-regulatory mechanisms prevent excessive temperature elevations above 41 °C. Temperatures > 38.3 °C are generally agreed as indicative of fever and should trigger further investigation
Hyperthermia	An unregulated rise in core temperature, where the mechanisms of regulation are damaged or overwhelmed. Temperature rises may be rapid and reach dangerously high levels
Hypothermia	A core body temperature < 35.0 °C. Hypothermia may occur inadvertently due to injury or exposure but may also be induced as a therapeutic measure in cardiac arrest or traumatic brain injury

Clinical Nursing Skills at a Glance, First Edition. Edited by Sarah Curr and Carol Fordham-Clarke.
© 2022 John Wiley & Sons Ltd. Published 2022 by John Wiley & Sons Ltd.
Companion website: www.wiley.com/go/clinicalnursingskills

Background

Thermoregulation is achieved through a balance of heat gain and heat loss. Heat is gained from metabolic activity, the functions of internal organs, and musculoskeletal activity. Heat is lost from the body by the four physical processes of conduction, convection, radiation, and evaporation (see Table 35.1).

The body's circadian rhythms create daily fluctuations, with temperature lowest in the morning and highest in the evening. Women have average temperatures higher than men due to the effect of menstrual hormonal regulation.

Core body temperature in humans is highly regulated and remains constant at 37°C (± 0.3°C). Core temperature is that of the blood circulating in the skull, thorax, and abdomen. Surface body temperature is highly variable. Non-invasive thermometers measure representations of core temperature at peripheral sites where core blood comes near to a body surface or orifice. Readings at these sites may be 0.5–1.5°C below that of core temperature. Temperature classifications are generally regarded as

- Normothermia: 37°C (± 0.3°C).
- Mild hypothermia: 32–35°C.
- Moderate hypothermia: 28–32°C.
- Severe hypothermia: 24–28 °C.
- Hyperthermia: ≥38°C.
- Hyperpyrexia: ≥40 °C.

(Monsieurs et al. 2015, Faulds and Meekings 2013):

Influencing Factors

- Hot or cold drinks and smoking affect oral temperatures for up to 15 minutes.
- An ear that has recently been placed against a pillow, exposed to cold air, or contains large amounts of ear wax may give inaccurate tympanic readings.
- Very thin patients may have an axillary pocket. A thermometer may not make contact with the chest wall and thus only read the air within this pocket.

Professional Approach

- Consider the most appropriate site for measurement.
- Explain the procedure fully, ensure understanding, and thus that consent is informed.

Equipment

- There are various instruments for taking the temperature non-invasively. Some are specific to one site, whereas others may be used in multiple sites.
- Tympanic spectrometry via the tympanic membrane of the ear.
- Electronic or digital thermometers for oral and axillary temperatures.
- Rectal electronic or digital thermometers.
- Disposable chemical dot thermometers for oral and axillary temperatures. These measure temperatures in the range of 35.5–40.4°C and are not suitable for detecting hypothermia or hyperpyrexia.
- Temporal arterial infrared spectrometry.

Procedure

- Perform hand hygiene and obtain informed consent.
- Prepare equipment – probe covers for tympanic thermometers must be used to prevent cross-infection. Electronic devices require regular calibrations (follow manufacturer's instructions).
- Check equipment is in good working order and the units of measurement and mode are set correctly. Chemical dot thermometers should be inspected for any inadvertent colour changes due to incorrect storage.
- Before taking the temperature, assess whether the patient's skin is cold and clammy or hot and sweaty.
- Use an appropriate site for taking the temperature. Avoid the oral site if the patient is unconscious or at risk of a seizure or biting the thermometer.
- Oral temperature is taken by inserting a suitable device into the left or right sublingual pocket of the mouth, located either side of the frenulum of the tongue. The patient should open their mouth and elevate the tongue. The probe is inserted into the pocket and the patient should close their lips around the probe or strip (Figure 35.1). Wait the appropriate amount of time according to manufacturer's instructions, before taking the reading and ensure that the last coloured dot is read when using a chemical thermometer (Figure 35.2).
- Tympanic temperature – follow the manufacturer's instructions. Using the thumb and index finger, take hold of the upper part of the pinna and pull upwards and backwards to perform an 'ear tug' (Figure 35.3). This straightens the ear canal, allowing a snug fit against the tympanic membrane.
- Axillary temperature – chemical dot thermometers can be used for axillary temperatures but will need to be held in place for three minutes. This site is the least accurate and should be avoided if other sites are available.
- Once a reading is obtained, dispose of the used strip or probe cover and store equipment appropriately.
- Interpret the result and document (Figure 35.4). Report any concerns (see Table 35.2).
- Temperature must form part of an overall assessment.

Red Flags

- Fever is an important part of the body's defence mechanisms and can be beneficial.
- Fever may be present without infection.
- If the device does not record, use an alternative with a range for hypo- and hyperthermia.
- Mercury-in-glass thermometers are no longer considered safe for clinical use, as mercury is a highly hazardous material.

References

Faulds, M. and Meekings, T. (2013). Temperature management in critically ill patients. *Continuing Education in Anaesthesia Critical Care & Pain* 13 (3): 75–79.

Monsieurs, K.G., Nolan, J.P., Bossaert, L.L. et al. (2015). European resuscitation council guidelines for resuscitation 2015 section 1. Executive summary. *Resuscitation* 95 (2015): 1–80.

36 Non-invasive circulatory assessment

Figure 36.1 (a, b) Changes in skin colour.

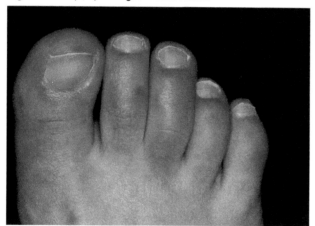

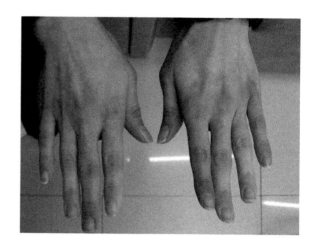

Figure 36.2 Blanching nail beds in capillary refill time.

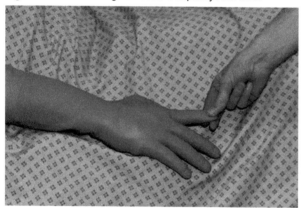

Figure 36.4 Sternum capillary refill time assessment.

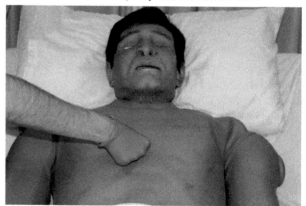

Figure 36.3 Documenting capillary refill time.

Changes in pulse, sensation and skin colour are late symptoms of neurovascular compromise (see front of chart for notes).	Neurovascular status	Pulse (with/ without doppler)	Present	●									
			Reduced in volume or rate since last assessment										
			Not present										
		Sensation	Normal	●									
			Abnormal/has changed from last assessment										
		Skin colour	Normal, responsive capillary refill	●									
			Pallor and/or slow/ absent capillary refill										
		Any abnormal neurovascular status observations should be escalated immediately											
			Initial	EX									

Background

An initial circulatory assessment will involve assessing level of consciousness and any new onset of confusion, measuring the respiratory rate, peripheral capillary oxygen saturation, pulse, blood pressure, temperature, capillary refill time (CRT), and inspection of the peripherals. This initial assessment gives an insight into the person's haemodynamic stability and whether care needs to be escalated (RCP 2017) for more intensive management.

Other circulatory assessment methods have been described within other chapters. Assessing the peripherals and CRT add to this assessment, are non-invasive, and are quick and easy to use.

Influencing Factors

- Exercise or other exerting activities within the last 15 minutes.
- Past medical history of peripheral vascular disease.
- Age-related factors.
- Ambient temperature.

Professional Approach

- Explain what you are doing and check understanding to ensure informed consent.
- Maintain privacy and dignity by minimising disturbances and closing the curtain or door.
- Ensure that any nail varnish is removed to enable visualisation of peripheral perfusion.
- Check for pain in the limbs and digits prior to performing assessment.

Equipment

- Equipment is not required for assessment of peripheral perfusion.
- A fob watch/watch with a second hand will be required for CRT measurement.

Procedure – Peripheral Assessment

- Visually inspect the lower legs, feet, and toes.
- Note the colour, e.g. pale, mottled, cyanosed (Figure 36.1) or red, flushed.
- Visually inspect the lower arms, hands, and fingers and note the colour.
- Touch toes, feet, and lower leg, noting if there is any change in temperature between the limbs.
- Note any heat, cold, clamminess, sweating.
- Repeat this in the lower arms, hands, and fingers.
- Document assessment and escalate any concerns.

Procedure – CRT

Applying pressure to the distal capillary bed obliterates blood flow and determines the time taken for blood flow to return. The CRT is indicative of the quality of perfusion and thus the patient's haemodynamic status:

- Hold the patient's hand above the level of the heart.
- Apply pressure to the digit for three to five seconds until complete blanching of the capillaries beneath is evident (Figure 36.2).
- Release pressure and monitor the time taken for colour and blood flow to return.
- Document (Figure 36.3).
- Escalate as appropriate, remembering that CRT is one measurement of the wider assessment.

NB: Remember that CRT can be assessed centrally over the sternum (Figure 36.4) but is usually peripherally on the nail bed of the fingers or toes.

Interpreting Results

- Cool, pale peripheries occur with vasoconstriction, poor perfusion, in low ambient temperature states, and with hypothermia. These are often indicative of circulatory distress, and treatment of the underlying cause needs to be commenced immediately.
- Warm peripheries and red and sweaty skin occur with vasodilatation and elevated body temperature. Increased core temperature can be indicative of an underlying infection.
- A normal CRT is < two seconds.
- A CRT > two seconds is indicative of poor perfusion.
- A CRT > five seconds implies an inadequate cardiac output and thus requires escalation and more intense management.

Red Flags

- Any change in perfusion between limbs could indicate an arterial occlusion, which is considered a vascular emergency.
- CRT is useful as an indicator of sepsis (Yasufumi et al. 2019) and if sepsis is suspected escalate and start the "sepsis six" pathway (NICE 2017).
- If you note any central cyanosis, (blue colour of skin and mucous membranes indicating poor oxygenation) this is a medical emergency and care must be escalated immediately.

References

National Institute of Health and Care Excellence (2017). *(NGS1) Sepsis: Recognition, Diagnosis, and Early Management*. London: National Institute of Health and Care Excellence.

Royal College of Physicians (2017). *National Early Warning Score (NEWS) 2*. London: Royal College of Physicians.

Yasufumi, O., Morimura, N., Shirasawa, A. et al. (2019). Quantitative capillary refill time predicts sepsis in patients with suspected infection in the emergency department: an observational study. *Journal of Intensive Care* 7 (29): 1–9.

37 Central venous pressure monitoring

Figure 37.1 Central venous catheter position.

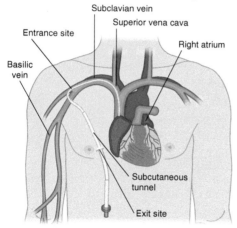

Figure 37.2 Pressure bag.

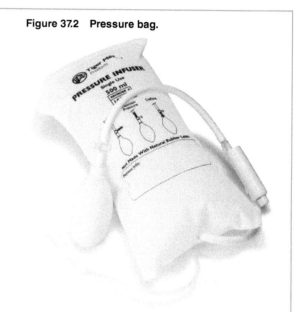

Figure 37.3 Identification of the phlebostatic axis.

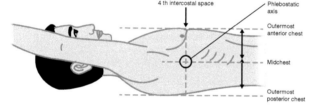

Figure 37.4 Central venous pressure waveform.

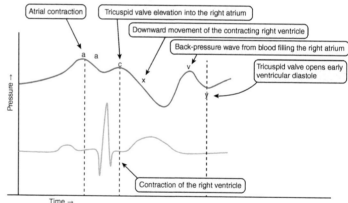

Figure 37.5 Trendelenburg position. *Source*: Redrawn from Nurselabs.com, 2020.

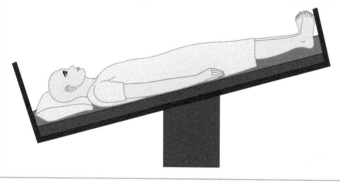

Clinical Nursing Skills at a Glance, First Edition. Edited by Sarah Curr and Carol Fordham-Clarke.
© 2022 John Wiley & Sons Ltd. Published 2022 by John Wiley & Sons Ltd.
Companion Website: www.wiley.com/go/clinicalnursingskills

Background

A central venous catheter (CVC) can be inserted into a central vein, commonly the subclavian or internal jugular, and then advanced to sit in the inferior vena cava, superior vena cava, or right atrium (Smith and Nolan 2018) (Figure 37.1). The CVC must sit in one of the above sites to ensure that it accurately measures the pressure in these areas (Hill 2018).

Although the CVC is often inserted to administer irritant medications that need to be delivered centrally or total parenteral nutrition, or is used when there is inadequate peripheral access (Sanfilippo et al. 2017), it is also used for haemodynamic monitoring. This monitoring largely occurs in the critically unwell patient to ensure adequate fluid resuscitation and maintenance (Sanfilippo et al. 2017). As such this chapter will focus on care of the CVC, its removal, and central venous pressure (CVP) monitoring.

Influencing Factors

Central venous catheter insertion and monitoring are indicated in the critically unwell adult but there are some instances where it is contraindicated:

- Infection at site.
- Major trauma affecting the site.
- Venous thrombosis or stenosis in intended vessel.
- Coagulopathy.
- Thrombocytopenia.

Professional Approach

- The healthcare professional must make the patient aware of the rationale for all procedures to obtain informed consent.
- The healthcare professional must be trained in all procedural elements prior to undertaking these to ensure patient safety.

Equipment – CVC Monitoring and Site Care

- Appropriate intravenous fluid and giving set.
- Pressure bag (Figure 37.2).
- Three-way tap and transducer.
- Monitor.
- Disposable apron and non-sterile gloves.

Procedure – CVP Monitoring

- Assess the pressure bag to ensure that it is set at 300 mmHg.
- Check the patency and date when the intravenous giving set was commenced to ensure it is changed every 72–96 hours (Loveday et al. 2014).
- Check the date of CVC insertion to ensure that it is changed every 7–10 days (Loveday et al. 2014).
- Examine the semi-permeable transparent dressing and assess site using VIP score.
- Ask the patient to lie flat, or at the angle of the previous CVP measurement, to ensure accuracy of results.
- Ensure that the patient is relaxed and breathing normally.
- Assess the transducer to ensure that it is taped at the phlebostatic axis (Figure 37.3).
- Select the CVP tab or section on the cardiac monitor.

NB: You must be trained on the monitor, and all medical devices, prior to use.

- Put on gloves and apron.
- Turn the three-way tap to open to air position, removing the cap as required.
- Press the CVP "zero" button on the monitor; you may need to hold it for a few seconds.
- Wait until the "zero" line appears.
- Turn the three-way tap to open to patient, replace the cap.
- Note the waveform and check for abnormalities (Figure 37.4).
- Note the numerical value. The normal range for CVP may vary but is usually considered to be between 3 and 6 cmH$_2$O.
- Remove gloves and apron and decontaminate hands.
- Document appropriately.
- Advise the patient of results where applicable.
- If required, support the patient into the preferred position.

Equipment – CVC Removal

- Wound dressing pack, including stitch cutter.
- Sterile gloves (if not medium).
- Sterile, occlusive dressing.
- Skin cleansing agent, i.e. 2% chlorhexidine in 70% isopropyl alcohol.
- Non-sterile gloves and disposable apron.
- Sterile specimen container (if appropriate).
- Sharps container.

Procedure – CVC Removal

- Decontaminate hands and apply gloves and apron.
- Clamp or disconnect any intravenous medications or fluids being administered via the CVC line.
- Prepare all equipment on a dressing trolley following steps outlined in Chapter 63.
- Lie the patient in the Trendelburg (Figure 37.5) position.
- Remove dressing and securing device if used.
- Place above, gloves and apron in clinical waste bag.
- Decontaminate hands, apply sterile gloves (Chapter 63).
- Clean site using appropriate cleansing agent.
- Instruct the patient to perform the Valsalva manoeuvre to reduce the risk of air entry. If the patient is ventilated, remove the CVC at the end expiration point.
- Place the gauze over the insertion point.
- Gently withdraw the CVC while applying firm pressure with the gauze.
- Maintain pressure for 5–10 minutes.
- Apply new dressing.
- Check the CVC tip is intact; send tip for culture if required.
- Ensure the patient stays in the supine position for a minimum of 30 minutes (Dougherty 2015).
- Document rationale for removal, date and time.

Red Flags

➤ An upright position for CVC removal can result in air embolism, as can leaving the CVC port open.

References

Dougherty, L. (2015). How to remove a non-tunnelled central venous catheter. *Nursing Standard* 30 (16–18): 36–39.

Hill, B.T. (2018). Role of central venous pressure monitoring in critical care settings. *Nursing Standard* 32 (23): 41–48.

Loveday, H., Wilson, J.A., Pratt, R. et al. (2014). epic3: National Evidence-Based Guidelines for preventing healthcare-associated infections in NHS hospitals in England. *Journal of Hospital Infection* 86: S1–S70.

Sanfilippo, F., Noto, A., Farbo, M. et al. (2017). Central venous pressure monitoring via peripherally or centrally inserted central catheters: a systematic review and meta-analysis. *The Journal of Vascular Access* 18 (4): 273–278.

Smith, R.N. and Nolan, J.P. (2018). Central venous catheters. *British Medical Journal* 2013 (347): 1–11.

38 Electrocardiogram

Figure 38.1 PQRST wave. *Source: Aaronson et al. (2012)/John Wiley & Sons.*

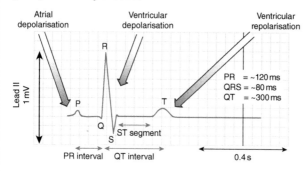

Figure 38.2 12-lead ECG placement. *Source: Aaronson et al. (2012)/John Wiley & Sons.*

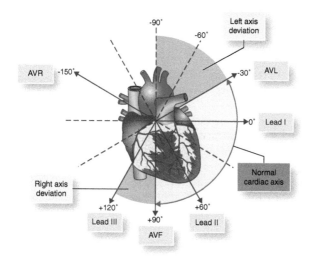

Figure 38.3 3-lead ECG.

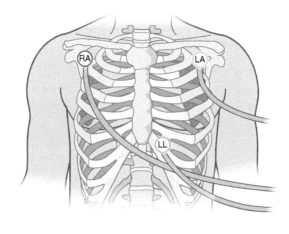

Figure 38.4 Eindhoven's triangle. *Source: Aaronson et al. (2012)/John Wiley & Sons.*

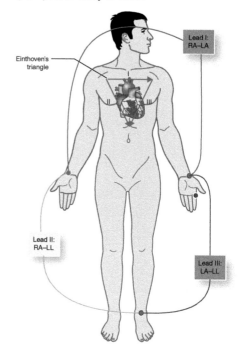

Figure 38.5 5-lead ECG.

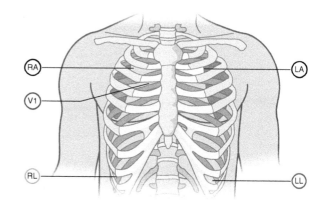

Table 38.1 Electrocardiogram (ECG) wave formation.

P	Depolarisation across atria
PR interval	Electrical conduction through the AV node
QRS	Depolarisation across the ventricles
T	Ventricular repolarisation

Once repolarisation is complete, the process will be repeated.

Background

The cardiac cycle consists of ventricular contraction (systole), ventricular relaxation (diastole), and ventricular filling. This cycle is stimulated by electrical activity within the cardiac muscle, the myocardium. These cells within the myocardium are joined together by their electrical connection. The contraction of one cell brings a rise in the cells' calcium concentration, which leads to depolarisation, and contraction across the myocardium. Although the heart rate is controlled by the cardiac centre, located within the brain stem, it is the sino-atrial node (SA), a group of cells within the right atrium, that controls heart contraction locally and it is here that the wave of depolarisation starts. As such, these cells are known as the pacemaker cells. The SA node fires to the atrioventricular (AV) node, and from the AV node the electrical impulse spreads through the bundle of His, sometimes referred to as the AV bundle. From the bundle of His, this wave of depolarisation spreads to the right and left branches and to the Purkinje fibres, which stimulate ventricular contraction. This activity is represented as a wave on the ECG recording (Figure 38.1; Table 38.1).

12-Lead Electrocardiogram (ECG)

A 12-lead ECG shows the electrical activity (Figure 38.2) from 12 different angles of the heart, whereas the 3-lead ECG (Figure 38.3), usually used for basic cardiac monitoring, only shows one view of the heart (commonly V2). In a 12-lead ECG there are six precordial chest leads and six limb leads. The chest leads are V1–V6 and they show:

- V1 – the right anterior (right atrium).
- V2 – the right anterior surface and some left anterior surface (left ventricle).
- V3 – the septum.
- V4 – the anterior surface of the left ventricle.
- V5 – the left anterior/left lateral surface of left ventricle.
- V6 – the left lateral aspect of left ventricle (Figure 38.4).

The six limb leads involve the placement of four electrodes: three from Einthoven's triangle (; Einthoven et al. 1950) with the fourth (N) stabilising the recording. This triangle generates six different views of the heart. The areas in these specific leads show:

- I – the left lateral aspect.
- II – the left lateral and inferior aspect.
- III – the interior surface.
- AVR – the right atrium.
- AVL – the left lateral surface.
- AVF – the inferior aspect.

Influencing Factors – ECG Indications

- As part of clinical screening.
- When patients present with palpitations.
- When there is a history of unexplained falls or syncope episodes.
- If any irregularity in the heart rate is noted, including tachycardia and bradycardia.

The graphic recording of heart activity provided by the ECG will highlight any heart disease or damage, or any problems with the heart conduction system, e.g. heart block.

Professional Approach

Before undertaking the ECG, explain why the procedure is being performed and obtain informed consent. To ensure privacy and dignity is maintained as much as possible, it is important to reduce the risk of interruptions and ensure that you have all your equipment.

Equipment

- A fully operational ECG machine with tracing paper.
- A minimum of 10 electrodes (useful to bring spares).
- A razor.
- Cleaning material.

Procedure

All electrodes should be placed in the correct position to ensure that an accurate recording is obtained. Once the electrodes are placed and leads attached, advise the patient to remain as still as possible and obtain your tracing. If artefact (interference on the recording) is present, it could be due to movement, the electrodes, or the actual ECG machine. If the electrodes are not sticking adequately it may be necessary to:

- shave the area in accordance with local Trust policy and patient consent.
- clean the area; particularly if oils or lotions have been applied.

If the ECG battery is low, it may be necessary to plug it into the mains while undertaking the tracing. If the patient is moving involuntarily, it may be that artefact remains and a note of this should be made and the healthcare professional interpreting the ECG notified.

Procedure – 3-Lead ECG/5-Lead ECG

In a 3-lead ECG there are three electrodes to be placed at the right shoulder (red), left shoulder (yellow), and left lower thoracic cage (green). A 5-lead ECG involves two additional electrodes to be placed at the right lower thoracic cage (black) and the V1 position (white). The 5-lead ECG (Figure 38.5) combines the lead II view with V1 to provide a left and a right view of the heart.

NB: Only those with appropriate training can read an ECG.

Red Flags

- If electrical activity is showing on the ECG but the patient has no pulse and is displaying no signs of life, pulseless electrical activity (PEA) should be expected. This is a cardiac arrest rhythm and should be treated with appropriate life support.

References

Aaronson, P.I., Ward, J.P.T., and Connolly, M.J. (2012). *The Cardiovascular System at a Glance*, 4e. John Wiley & Sons.

Einthoven W., Fahr G., & de Waart A. (1950) On the direction and manifest size of the variations of potential in the human heart and on the influence of the position of the heart on the form of the electrocardiogram. *American. Heart Journal.* 40 (2) 163–211. (Reprint 1913, translated by THE Hoff, P Sekelj).

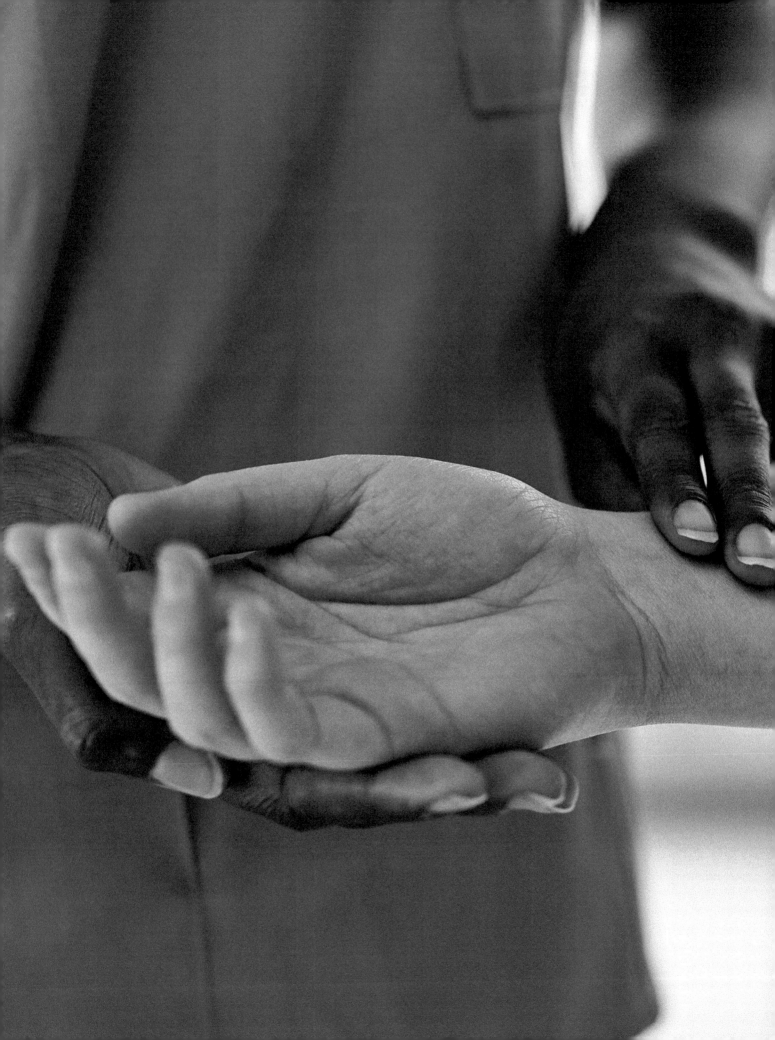

Gastrointestinal skills

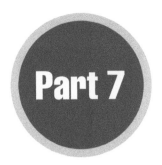

Part 7

Chapters

39 Nutritional screening

Figure 39.1   Stadiometer.

(a)
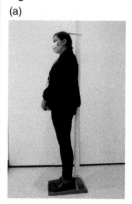

(b)
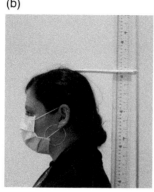

Figure 39.2   Weighing scales.
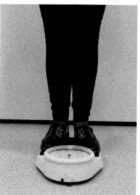

Figure 39.3   Estimating height from ulna length. *Source: The 'MUST' Explanatory Booklet/BAPEN.*
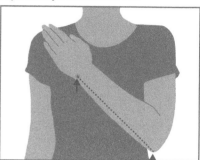

Figure 39.4   Estimating body mass index (BMI) category from mid upper arm circumference (MUAC). *Source: The 'MUST' Explanatory Booklet/BAPEN.*

Estimating BMI category from mid upper arm circumference (MUAC)

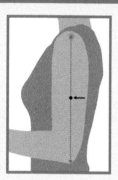

The subject's left arm should be bent at the elbow at a 90 degree angle, with the upper arm held parallel to the side of the body. Measure the distance between the bony protrusion on the shoulder (acromion) and the point of the elbow (olecranon process). Mark the mid-point.

Ask the subject to let arm hang loose and measure around the upper arm at the mid-point, making sure that the tape measure is snug but not tight.

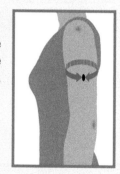

If MUAC is <23.5 cm, BMI is likely to be <20 kg/m².
If MUAC is >32.0 cm, BMI is likely to be >30 kg/m².

The use of MUAC provides a general indication of BMI and is not designed to generate an actual score for use with 'MUST'. For further information on use of MUAC please refer to *The 'MUST' Explanatory Booklet.*

Background

Malnutrition has long been a concern to health and well-being, impeding recovery and increasing the risk of mortality after an adverse event (McEvilly 2016). It also brings a cost of £23.5bn to healthcare across the UK (Stratton et al. 2018), and reducing it is a key part of any baseline assessment.

This nutritional screening identifies individuals at risk of malnutrition. If an individual is found to be at risk of malnutrition upon assessment, a referral to a dietician or nutritional nurse specialist for a more detailed nutritional assessment occurs.

Influencing Factors

- Many factors can affect nutritional status and the underlying cause needs to be established to ensure appropriate treatment can be commenced.
- When measuring weight, it is important to do this at the same time every day for consistency and accuracy of the results.
- For some patients, the weight may not be reflective of their body mass index (BMI), e.g. in cases of amputation, and thus alternative methods will need to be used.

Professional Approach

- Ensure that the rationale for the screening process and subsequent actions are fully explained to the patient.
- Ensure that you have received the necessary training to complete the assessment competently.

Equipment

- The Malnutrition Universal Screening Tool (MUST) tool (BAPEN 2011) or any other locally used nutritional assessment.
- Stadiometer (Figure 39.1).
- Clinical scales (Figure 39.2).

Procedure – Initial Assessment

Discussion with the patient may include the following:

- Usual eating patterns – e.g. how many meals eaten per day; at what times; who with; how much of each meal is eaten?
- Recognising any recent changes in dietary intake – e.g. loss of appetite, changes in ability to meet nutritional needs, taste changes?
- Recent weight loss – remember to ask if this was intentional.
- Ability to eat and drink – e.g. are there any factors that limit this; do they need assistance; is this assistance available?
- Gastrointestinal factors – e.g. reflux, nausea and vomiting or change in bowel habit.
- Ability to access food or fluid – e.g. mobility, ability to prepare food; who shops for food and how often?
- Oral assessment – e.g. oral discomfort, rotten or missing teeth, ill-fitting or broken dentures.
- Identifying psychological factors – depression or loneliness can have an impact on appetite or motivation to eat and drink.

The following observations may suggest potential malnutrition:

- Clothes or jewellery, particularly rings, may be loose-fitting.
- Dentures may be ill-fitting.
- Skin may appear dry with reduced elasticity.
- Oedema.

These observations are important when considering an individual with cognitive impairment who may not be able to respond to the questions above.

Procedure – the MUST Tool

The MUST is recommended by NICE (2017) and is commonly used throughout the UK (BAPEN 2011). It is a five-step screening tool that identifies adults who are malnourished, at risk of becoming malnourished, or obese.

Step 1: BMI score

When measuring height and weight, BAPEN recommend that a stadiometer and clinical scales are used where possible (Figures 39.1a and 39.1b). Shoes should be removed for both weight and height. The BMI can then be calculated using the formula below or using a BMI chart.

$$BMI = \frac{Weight\,(kg)}{Height\,(m^2)}$$

If measurements cannot be taken, then the patient can self-report. If this is not feasible alternative measurements can be used:

- Estimating height from ulna length (Figure 39.3).
- Estimating BMI category from mid upper arm circumference (MUAC) (Figure 39.4). This is not recommended if oedema is present.

Data collected can be compared to charts from BAPEN.

Step 2: Weight loss score

Unintentional weight loss in the last 3–6 months is scored.

If neither BMI nor weight loss can be determined, BAPEN (2011) recommends the use of the following subjective criteria:

- BMI – Is the individual thin, an acceptable weight or overweight?
- Weight loss – Have the individual's clothes or jewellery become loose-fitting; has food intake decreased for any reason over the last three to six months; are there underlying disease or psychosocial/physical issues that may have caused weight loss?

Step 3: Acute disease effect

Is the patient acutely unwell with little or no nutritional intake for more than five days?

This score is more likely to affect in-patients than those in the out-patient or community setting.

Step 4: Overall risk of malnutrition

Adding the scores of steps 1–3 together will give an overall risk of malnutrition – low, medium or high.

Step 5: Management guidelines

Both MUST management guidelines and local policy can be used to develop an appropriate individualised plan of the care for the individual being assessed.

Red Flags

- It is important to remember that an obese individual can still be malnourished.

References

BAPEN (2011) *The 'MUST' Explanatory Booklet.* www.bapen.org.uk/pdfs/must/must_explan.pdf (accessed 13 October 2020).

McEvilly, A. (2016). Identifying and managing malnutrition. *British Journal of Community Nursing.* 21 (S7): S14–S21.

NICE (2017). *Nutrition Support for Adults: Oral Nutrition Support, Enteral Tube Feeding and Parental Nutrition.* London: NICE.

Stratton, R., Smith, T., and Gabe, S. (2018). *Managing Malnutrition to Improve Lives and Save Money.* BAPEN: Redditch.

40 Supporting eating and drinking

Table 40.1 Example of food chart.

Surname.......... Stanner........................
First name........ Elizabeth......................
D.O.B........... 27.02.46 ....
Hospital ...... C2469T.............................

FOOD INTAKE CHART

Date...14.10.17...... Weight...48kg..........
BMI...17.8............ Height....1.64m........

Please record everything eaten throughout the day. Please record what is actually eaten not the portion offered. Eg. 1 tablespoon carrots, 2 slices wholemeal bread, 1 medium potato

	DAY 1 Date	DAY 2 Date
Breakfast	2 tablespoons porridge 1 teaspoon sugar	
Mid morning	2 chocolate biscuits	
Lunch	2 small potatoes 1 tablespoon peas 1 tablespoon beef stew	
Mid afternoon	2 chocolate biscuits	
Evening meal		
Evening and during night		

Figure 40.1   Red tray.

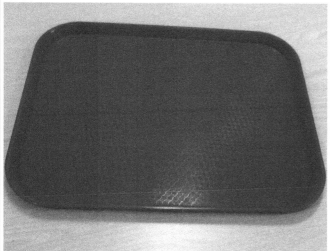

Figure 40.2   Adapted cutlery.

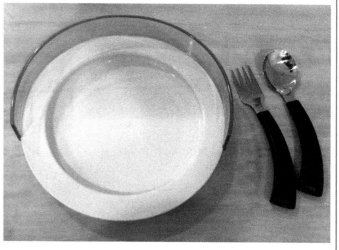

Clinical Nursing Skills at a Glance, First Edition. Edited by Sarah Curr and Carol Fordham-Clarke.
© 2022 John Wiley & Sons Ltd. Published 2022 by John Wiley & Sons Ltd.
Companion website: www.wiley.com/go/clinicalnursingskills

Background

For many people, mealtimes are about more than just food. Location, company, and comfort all play a part in how individuals feel about eating, which is essentially a social as well as an essential experience.

Influencing Factors

There are many factors that can affect eating and drinking. Below are some of those to be considered when supporting eating and drinking in the healthcare setting:

- Food allergies.
- Religious or cultural requirements.
- Food preferences.
- Presentation.
- Portion size.
- Level of support required.
- Availability of adapted cutlery and crockery.
- Comfort.
- Use of toilet beforehand.
- Pain or nausea.
- Environment – by bed or communal day room.
- Urinals, waste nearby.

Professional Approach

- Consider whether you have the time to support eating and drinking.
- Ensure that you read the care plan and that you are aware of the support required.
- Document actions taken and food and drink ingested, if required, after completion (Table 40.1).

Professional Approach – Strategies to Support Eating and Drinking

Modification of Food and Fluids

- Assist patient in choosing food from menu.
- Consider special diets.
- Assess ability to chew and swallow.
- Determine if soft or puréed diets are required.

Swallowing Strategies

- Liaise with the speech and language team (SALT).
- Prompted swallowing or individualised swallowing techniques may be recommended.
- Patients should be encouraged and supported to practise these techniques.

Protected Mealtimes

These were developed to combat the malnutrition that occurs in the in hospital environment (Porter, Ottrey, & Huggins, 2017). Protected mealtimes provide a quiet uninterrupted environment at mealtimes facilitates patients' nutritional intake by enabling healthcare workers and relatives to help patients with eating and drinking.

The Use of Red Trays (Figure 40.1)

This highlights vulnerable patients who may need support with eating and drinking (Bradley & Rees 2003).

Preparation

- Patients may need support to sit upright, in order to prevent aspiration.
- Ensure tables are within easy reach of the patient and at the correct height.
- Plates and cutlery need to be positioned so that patients with visual impairments can see or access them.

- Consider use of supportive cutlery and crockery (Figure 40.2).
- Offer snacks if patient will not sit for meals.
- Consider strategies for cognitively impaired patients, e.g. involving carers, identifying favourite foods.
- Obtain informed consent.
- Consider and respect privacy and dignity.
- Support patients to maintain independence.

NB: The provision of nutritional support is not always appropriate. This is a decision that should be made as a team, including the patient and their family members and carers.

Equipment

This may include:

- A red tray.
- Adapted cutlery and/or crockery.
- Chair (for you to sit on; this is easily forgotten in a busy environment).

Procedure – Feeding an Adult Patient

- Assist the patient to sit upright, preferably out of bed.
- Ensure that the patient is comfortable and has clean hands and mouth, including teeth or dentures (if applicable).
- Ask if they would like to visit the toilet.
- Wash your hands.
- Position yourself so that the patient can see you, considering any visual impairment.
- Sit down to indicate you have time to support their eating and drinking.
- If appropriate ask the patient how they would prefer food to be offered: e.g. one flavour at a time; with condiments, sauces or gravy; using a spoon or fork.
- Otherwise, observe the patient's non-verbal communication and respond to this.
- Allow the patient to finish each mouthful before offering another.
- Observe for coughing or choking. If the patient appears to be having difficulty in swallowing, stop feeding immediately and refer to SALT. This may be indicated by dribbling.
- Judge whether the patient would like to engage in conversation during meals. Try to avoid asking questions when they have their mouth full.
- Offer regular sips of drink during the meal.
- If the patient does not appear to be enjoying the meal, offer an alternative or move on to the next course.
- After eating, assist the patient to clean their face and hands. Ask if they would like to brush their teeth or use a mouthwash.
- Document what the patient has eaten, as required.
- Complete fluid balance chart, as required.

Red Flags

- Patients who present with recurrent chest infections may have underlying swallowing issues and should be assessed by SALT.
- Patients with a reduced level of consciousness should not be fed orally as they are at risk of aspiration.

References

Bradley, L. & Rees, C. (2003) Reducing nutritional risk in hospital: the red tray. *Nursing Standard*. 17 (26), 33–37.

Porter, J., Ottrey, E. & Huggins, C.E. (2017) Protected mealtimes in hospitals and nutritional intake: systematic review and meta-analyses. *International Journal of Nursing Studies* 65 (2017), 62–69

41 Nasogastric tube insertion

Figure 41.1   Fine-bore tube.

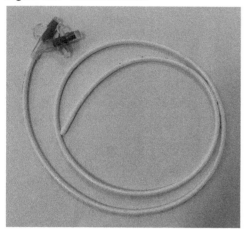

Figure 41.2   Large bore tube

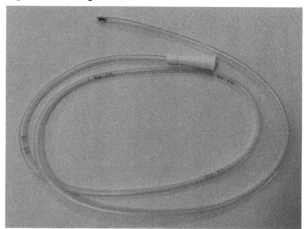

Figure 41.3   Nose to ear to xiphisternum (NEX) measurement

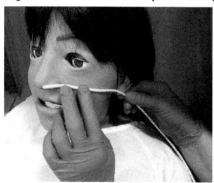
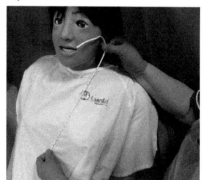

Figure 41.4   Obtaining gastric aspirate.

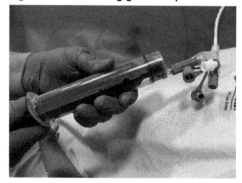
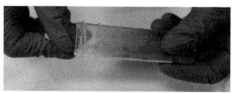

Figure 41.5   Assessing gastric pH.

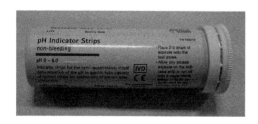
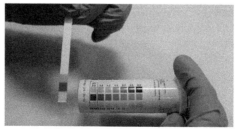

Clinical Nursing Skills at a Glance, First Edition. Edited by Sarah Curr and Carol Fordham-Clarke.
© 2022 John Wiley & Sons Ltd. Published 2022 by John Wiley & Sons Ltd.
Companion website: www.wiley.com/go/clinicalnursingskills

Background

A nasogastric tube is inserted through the nose into the stomach via the oesophagus. A fine-bore nasogastric feeding tube may be used for short-term nutritional support. A wide-bore nasogastric tube can be used for drainage or aspiration of gastric fluid or air, or for stomach lavage.

Influencing Factors

In some circumstances, nasogastric tube insertion is not appropriate. These include:

- Severe facial trauma.
- Recent nasal surgery.
- Abnormal clotting.
- Oesophageal varices or fistulae.
- Oesophageal pouch.
- Basal skull fracture.
- Non-functioning gastrointestinal tract (NNNG 2016).

Professional Approach

- Ensure that you obtain informed consent by explaining the rationale for the procedure.
- Accept the client's right to refuse, but explore any refusal to understand the patient's fears or concerns.
- Be sensitive to the psychological impact of having a highly visible feeding tube.
- Provide education for ongoing care to the client and their family members or carers.
- Remember that you have ongoing accountability for confirming that the tube is in the stomach.

Equipment

- Nasogastric tube appropriate for intended purpose and in accordance with local policy (Figures 41.1 and 41.2).
- Non-sterile gloves and apron and other PPE if appropriate.
- 50 mL purple enteral syringe.
- pH indicator strips (CE marked for human aspirate).
- Receiver or vomit bowl.
- Tissues.
- Hypoallergenic tape and scissors or specific nasogastric retention device or dressing.
- Water for flushing (as per local policy).
- Glass of water with drinking straw, if appropriate.

Procedure

- Explain and discuss the procedure with the patient to obtain informed consent.
- Agree a signal that means "stop" as part of this conversation.
- Assist the patient to sit in a semi-upright position, if possible.
- Complete NEX measurement (nose to ear to xiphisternum; Figure 41.3) using either a tape measure or the tube itself (this estimates the approximate length of the tube to be inserted).
- Check nostril patency by asking the patient to sniff through each nostril while occluding the other.
- Wash hands and put on gloves and apron, and a mask and visor as appropriate.
- Lubricate tube as per manufacturer's recommendations.
- Insert the tube into the chosen nostril, sliding it along the floor of the nasal passage horizontally.

- When the tube reaches the nasopharynx, some resistance will be felt. If appropriate, ask the patient to take a sip of water and swallow. Advance tube with each swallow.
- Gently advance the tube until it reaches the predetermined NEX measurement.
- If the patient shows signs of respiratory distress, stop and remove the tube.
- Secure the tube as per manufacturer's recommendations or local policy.
- Using a 50 mL enteral syringe, draw back on the tube to obtain gastric aspirate (Figure 41.4).
- Test pH of aspirate using CE marked indicator strips (NHS Improvement 2016) (Figure 41.5).
- Do not remove the introducer (if used) until correct placement has been confirmed according to local policy.
- Dispose of waste according to standard precautions.
- Document procedure as per local guidelines. This should include reason for insertion, type of tube used, how long it can stay in situ, length of tube inserted, and pH of aspirate.

Procedure – Checking Tube Placement

- Local policy must be followed when checking tube placement immediately post-insertion; this may be via X-ray or pH of aspiration.
- Confirm tube length.
- Repeat placement checks:
  - before administering each feed.
  - before giving medication.
  - after extensive coughing or physiotherapy.
  - at least once daily.

Procedure – If Unable to Gain Aspirate

- Turn patient onto left side.
- Inject 10–20 mL air into tube using a 50 mL enteral syringe.
- Wait 15–30 minutes before aspirating again.
- Advance/withdraw tube by 10–20 cm.
- Give oral hygiene to stimulate gastric secretions.
- Do not flush with water until position ascertained (NNNG 2016).

Red Flags

- Do not administer anything down the tube until correct placement has been confirmed by a pH < 5.5 (NHS Improvement 2016).
- Shortness of breath and/or severe pain could indicate damage to the lung, and care must be escalated to ensure correct management.
- If using a guidewire, never reinsert while the tube remains in the patient.

References

NEW National Nurses Nutrition Group (NNNG) (2016) *Safe Insertion and Ongoing Care of Nasogastric (NG) Feeding Tubes in Adults.* www.nnng.org.uk/wp-content/uploads/2016/06/NNNG-Nasogastric-tube-Insertion-and-Ongoing-Care-Practice-Final-Aprill-2016.pdf (accessed 30 November 2020).

NHS Improvement (2016). *Patient Safety Alert: Nasogastric Tube Misplacement: Risk of Death and Severe Harm Through Failure to Implement Previous Guidance.* London: NHS Improvement.

42 Enteral feeding

Figure 42.1 Gastrotomy tube.

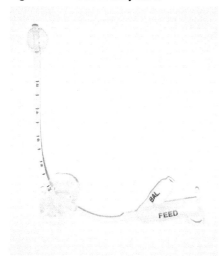

Figure 42.2 Oral syringes.

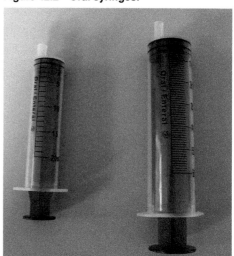

Figure 42.3 Enteral feeding.

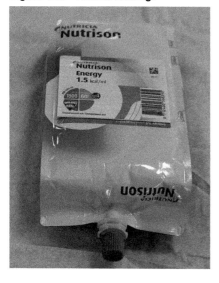

Figure 42.4 Enteral feeding equipment.

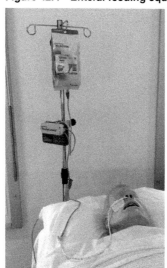

Figure 42.5 Liquid medication.

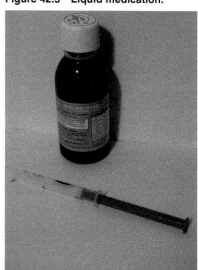

Clinical Nursing Skills at a Glance, First Edition. Edited by Sarah Curr and Carol Fordham-Clarke.
© 2022 John Wiley & Sons Ltd. Published 2022 by John Wiley & Sons Ltd.
Companion website: www.wiley.com/go/clinicalnursingskills

Background

If patients are unable to tolerate feeding directly into the stomach, alternative feeding tubes can be used:

- Nasoduodenal.
- Nasojejunal.
- Gastrostomy.
- Jejunostomy.

These tubes are usually inserted endoscopically or in radiology to ensure correct positioning.

- A percutaneous endoscopic gastrostomy (PEG) (Figure 42.1) tube is inserted via the abdominal wall and held in place with an internal balloon or bumper and an external fixator.
- A percutaneous endoscopic jejunostomy (PEJ) tube is inserted into the jejunum via the abdominal wall.
- A radiological inserted gastrostomy (RIG) tube refers to the method of insertion.

Influencing Factors

- The correct syringe size must be used, a purple syringe between 30 and 50 mL, as smaller syringes may create higher pressure and thus damage to the tube.
- Flush with 15–30 mL of water but refer to local policy on whether sterile water or tap water is preferred.
- Use sterile water for jejunal tubes as the stomach and gastric juice are bypassed.

Professional Approach

- Explain what you are doing and why to obtain informed consent.
- Be mindful of the patient's privacy requirements. This may also include a request for an alternative member of staff.

Equipment – Flushing Feeding Tube

- 50 mL oral syringe (Figure 42.2).
- Sterile or tap water.

Procedure – Flushing Feeding Tubes

- This is essential to avoid tube blockage and should occur:
  - before and after medication.
  - before and after feed administration.
- Draw up the required amount of water in the appropriate syringe.
- Check the site for signs of infection.
- Close the clamp on the feeding infusion set, if being provided, and remove the feeding infusion set from the port.
- Attach the syringe to the port and use a pulsatile action to create turbulence within the lumen of the feeding tube (Pickering 2015).
- Flush with 15–30 mL of water but refer to local policy on whether sterile water or tap water is preferred.
- Once flushed, continue with the procedure which may include enteral feeding or medication administration.
- Document all actions once complete.
- Refer to dietician or nutrition nurse specialist for further guidance.

Equipment – Administering Feed or Flush via Enteral Feeding Tube

- Sterile water, tap water, or enteral feed (Figures 42.3 and 42.4).
- Feeding infusion set.
- Oral syringe (Figure 42.2).

Procedure for Administration of Feed or Flush Via Enteral Feeding Tube

- Discuss procedure with patient and obtain informed consent.
- Check feed against prescription, the expiry date, that the seal is not broken, and the appearance of the feed to ensure that it has not curdled.
- Calculate rate, if not stipulated on prescription.
- Wash hands and put on gloves and apron.
- Ascertain position of tube prior to use.
- Ensure patient is sitting at a 35° angle or greater to reduce the risk of aspiration. Ensure that they remain at this angle throughout the feed and for 30 minutes post-feed.
- Remove cap from feed and pierce film with sterile infusion set using aseptic non-touch technique (ANTT).
- Close roller clamp, if available, and hang feed onto infusion set.
- Prime infusion set as per manufacturer's instructions. Ensure that you are trained and competent to use the pump.
- Attach giving set to pump and set pump as per manufacturer's instructions.
- Set dose so that the pump will alarm on feed completion. This allows you to respond to the alarm and take appropriate action, thus reducing the risk of tube blockage.
- Draw up 15–30 mL of water in a 50 mL purple syringe.
- Attach the syringe to the tube port, ensuring any other ports are closed, and flush using a pulsatile action.
- Attach the primed set to the feeding tube port and start the feed, ensuring that roller clamps are open.
- Dispose of waste according to standard precautions.
- Document as per local policy.

Procedure – Administering Medication via Enteral Feeding Tube

- Consider if another method of administration can be used.
- Liaise with medical team to ensure minimum necessary medication is prescribed and that it is prescribed for the correct route.
- Discuss appropriate medication formulations for enteral tube administration with dietician or nutrition nurse specialist and pharmacist. Oral medication is prescribed and may come ready to be administered (Figure 42.5) but may require some preparation. Do not crush medications for administration. Tube type and size will have an impact on which formulation should be used.
- Medication should not be added directly into enteral feed. Feed should be stopped prior to medication administration and the tube should be flushed.
- Each medication should be administered separately, and the tube should be flushed with water between medications to reduce the risk of compatibility issues. Refer to local policy for volume of flush.
- If medication is prepared in a separate pot, the pot should be rinsed with water after the medication has been delivered and then this rinsing fluid should be administered to ensure that all medication has been delivered (White 2015.)

Red Flags

- ☛ Document tube length and pH of gastric aspirate for nasogastric tubes before feeding/flushing or adding medication.
- ☛ Some medication may not be licensed to be administered via an enteral tube.

References

Pickering, K. (2015). Flushing enteral feeding tubes. In: *Handbook of Drug Administration Via Enteral Feeding Tubes. Third Edition* (eds. R. White and V. Bradnam), 70–87. London. Pharmaceutical Press.

White, R. (2015). Choice of medication formulation. In: *Handbook of Drug Administration Via Enteral Feeding Tubes*, 3e (eds. R. White and V. Bradnam), 115–150. London. Pharmaceutical Press.

43 Management of diarrhoea

Table 43.1 Classification of diarrhoea.

Classification	Explanation
Osmotic	Too much water is drawn into the bowel, e.g. malabsorption.
Secretary	Increased secretion of fluid and electrolytes and decreased absorption, e.g. infection.
Inflammatory	Damaged mucosal cells, e.g. ulcerative colitis.
Abnormal gut motility	Increased motility.

Source: Based on World Gastroenterology Organisation (2012).

Table 43.2 Nursing management of diarrhoea.

Intervention	Rationale
Infection control	A risk assessment should be carried out to determine whether the patient needs to be in isolation or not. Decontaminate hands with soap and water as alcohol hand gels are ineffective against some infections causing diarrhoea.
Comfort	Anti-spasmodic drugs may be useful to ease cramping but should only be used following discussion with the medical team.
Skin integrity	Frequent diarrhoea can cause anal or perianal discomfort, particularly if the patient is incontinent of faeces. Skin cleansing and the use of moisturiser and/or a barrier cream following episodes of diarrhoea can reduce the risk of skin breakdown. Wipes are available that cleanse, moisturise, and protect the skin. The patient's skin should be monitored closely for evidence of incontinence (Baadjies et al. 2014).
Hydration and nutrition	Patient may have associated loss of appetite. Alternatively, they may fear eating or drinking in case it results in further diarrhoea. Maintenance of fluid balance and food charts alongside a stool chart may help determine whether the patient is at risk of dehydration or malnutrition.
Sleep disturbance	Diarrhoea may disturb sleep, resulting in fatigue. If anti-motility drugs are appropriate, they may allow the patient longer periods of rest and sleep between episodes of diarrhoea.
Psychological	It is essential that both privacy and dignity are maintained while caring for a patient with diarrhoea but ongoing diarrhoea can be isolating particularly if symptoms limit the individual's ability to carry out the activities of daily living. Monitor the psychological impact of diarrhoea on the patient.

Figure 43.1 Bristol Stool Chart. *Source*: Based on Wikimedia Commons, 2020.

Bristol Stool Chart

Type 1	Separate hard lumps, like nuts (hard to pass)
Type 2	Sausage-shaped but lumpy
Type 3	Like a sausage but with cracks on the surface
Type 4	Like a sausage or snake, smooth and soft
Type 5	Soft blobs with clear-cut edges
Type 6	Fluffy pieces with ragged edges, a mushy stool
Type 7	Watery, no solid pieces. Entirely Liquid

Figure 43.2 Skin integrity assessment.

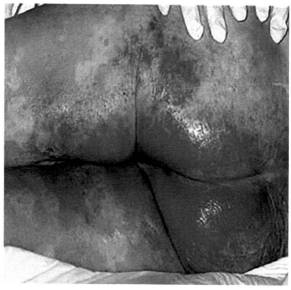

Clinical Nursing Skills at a Glance, First Edition. Edited by Sarah Curr and Carol Fordham-Clarke.
© 2022 John Wiley & Sons Ltd. Published 2022 by John Wiley & Sons Ltd.
Companion website: www.wiley.com/go/clinicalnursingskills

Background

The large intestine is where water is absorbed, and digested food is converted into faeces. It is divided up into four regions: the caecum, the colon, the rectum, and the anal canal. Immediately after a meal, peristalsis forces material from the ileum (small intestine) into the caecum. This material then travels through the colon to the rectum. As a result of water absorption, this material becomes solid and is now called faeces. The rectum stores faecal matter prior to expulsion via the anus. An internal sphincter prevents involuntary expulsion of faeces and an external sphincter, under voluntary control, can open and close to allow for the passage of faeces out through the anus.

Definition of Diarrhoea

Diarrhoea can be clinically classified as either:

- Acute – sudden-onset diarrhoea lasting less than four weeks; usually self-limiting.
- Chronic – diarrhoea that lasts longer than four weeks and may require further investigation (WGO 2012) (Table 43.1).

Influencing Factors – Pharmacological Interventions

The overarching aim here is to prevent dehydration. This may well be achieved through:

- Oral rehydration solutions (ORS).
- Intravenous infusion and electrolyte replacement (in more severe diarrhoea).
- Anti-motility drugs, to prolong the duration of intestinal transit.
- Anti-motility drugs used alongside an antibacterial – this may be of benefit in terms of patient comfort but should be discussed with the patient's medical team (Koo et al. 2009).
- Bulk-forming drugs, which may be useful in diverticular disease (BNF 2020).

Professional Approach

- If in a secondary care setting ensure that the patient has easy access to the toilet and mobility aids as needed.
- Each bowel motion will need to be measured and written on the fluid balance chart. Considering the patient's privacy and dignity needs will be essential here.

Equipment

- Assessment chart.
- Stool sample pot.
- Toileting aids.
- Bowel chart.

Procedure – Assessment

The aim of this assessment is to identify the most likely cause(s) of diarrhoea to develop an individualised plan of care. Assessment can include:

- Asking when did the diarrhoea start and were there any causative factors?
- Establishing if there has been previous gastrointestinal surgery.
- A description of stool and volume (Figure 43.1). Is there any blood or mucus? Is the stool fatty (ask if it floats)?
- Obtaining information on frequency and urgency of diarrhoea and timing, e.g. straight after meals or medication, at night.
- Questioning if there has been faecal incontinence.
- Asking about any associated symptoms, e.g. fever, pain, nausea, weight loss.
- Establishing general health, including psychological factors, e.g. stress.
- Considering what has worked in the past, if relevant.
- Receiving details on current medication and recent dose or medication changes.
- Establishing the impact of the diarrhoea on quality of life.
- Establishing impact on skin integrity (Figure 43.2) and providing appropriate treatment (Baadjies et al. 2014).
- Requesting a stool specimen to send for cultures and sensitivity.

Red Flags

- ☛ Remember infection control measures when caring for patients with diarrhoea.
- ☛ Patients may be isolated and *Clostridium difficile* or *Noravirus* suspected. Use soap and water for hand decontamination in preference to alcohol hand gel (PHE 2013).
- ☛ Anti-motility drugs, for use during episodes of infectious diarrhoea, are discouraged.

N.B. After nursing assessment has been completed the nursing care planning, goals and interventions need to be commenced. Table 43.2 outlines some nursing and medical care that may be initiated.

References

Baadjies, R., Karrouze, I., and Rajpaul, K. (2014). Using no-rinse skin wipes to treat incontinence-associated dermatitis. *British Journal of Nursing* 23 (Sup20): S22–S28.

British National Formulary (2020) *Diarrhoea (Acute)*. https://bnf.nice.org.uk/treatment-summary/diarrhoea-acute.html (accessed 16 October 2020).

Koo, H., Koo, D., Musher, D., and DuPont, H. (2009). Antimotility agents for the treatment of clostridium difficile diarrhoea and colitis. *Clinical Infectious Diseases* 48 (5): 598–605.

Public Health England (2013). *Updated guidance on the management and treatment of Clostridium difficile infection*. London, Public Health England.

World Gastroenterology Organisation (2012). *Practice Guideline: Acute Diarrhoea*. Munich, Germany: WGO.

44 Management of constipation

Table 44.1 Factors influencing constipation.

Factor	Rationale
Gender	Women are more at risk than men
Age	Increased prevalence in older patients
Reduced mobility	• Reduced abdominal muscle activity affecting ease of defecation • To access the toilet independently
Fibre intake	• Change in appetite • Nil by mouth status • Limited availability of fibre-rich foods
Fluid intake	• Access to fluids • Reduced dexterity • Clinical dehydration
Environmental	• Change in routine • Lack of privacy • Use of a bedpan or commode rather than a toilet
Physiological	• Organic causes • Cognitive impairment
Psychological	• Depression • Anxiety
Medication	• Drug-induced • Laxative abuse

Table 44.2 Pharmacological interventions to reduce constipation.

Medication	Action
Bulk-forming laxatives	To increase faecal mass Not to be used in faecal impaction
Stimulant laxatives	To stimulate peristalsis and mucus secretion Not to be used in intestinal obstruction
Osmotic laxatives	Retain fluid in the bowel through osmosis
Stool softeners	Allow infiltration of water and fat into stools making defecation easier

Figure 44.2 When listening to the bowel, move systematically around all four quadrants of the abdomen.

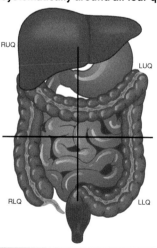

Figure 44.1 Correct position for opening your bowels.

Positions for defecation

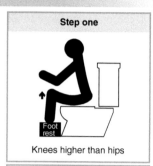

Step one

Knees higher than hips

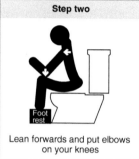

Step two

Lean forwards and put elbows on your knees

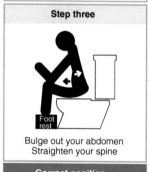

Step three

Bulge out your abdomen
Straighten your spine

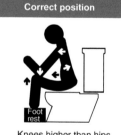

Correct position

Knees higher than hips
Lean forwards and put elbows on your knees
Bulge out your abdomen
Straighten your spine

Clinical Nursing Skills at a Glance, First Edition. Edited by Sarah Curr and Carol Fordham-Clarke.
© 2022 John Wiley & Sons Ltd. Published 2022 by John Wiley & Sons Ltd.
Companion website: www.wiley.com/go/clinicalnursingskills

Background

Constipation is a highly subjective condition with many causative factors. As a result, the condition tends to be defined in terms of symptoms. Our main aims are to prevent constipation from occurring and to provide relief if it does. Constipation can be clinically classified into three categories but may result from factors relating to more than one category:

- Primary/functional – associated with lifestyle factors with no pathophysiological cause.
- Secondary/organic – associated with an underlying pathology or condition affecting the bowel.
- Iatrogenic – constipation resulting from medication or treatment.

Influencing Factors

Factors influencing constipation are shown in Table 44.1.

Professional Approach

- Fully explain what the assessment involves and ensure that the patient is comfortable and consents with you proceeding.
- Make sure that you have enough time and that the patient does not have procedures or visitors scheduled.
- Maintain privacy and dignity and consider cultural and religious preferences.

Equipment

Ensure you are using appropriate assessment tools in accordance with local Trust policy.

Procedure – Assessment

The aim of assessment is to identify the probable cause(s) of constipation to develop an individualised plan of care and prevent recurrence. Assessment may include:

- Description of symptoms.
- Description of stool. Refer to Bristol Stool Chart. (Figure 43.1)
- Frequency of normal and current bowel habit.
- Change in bowel habit – identify possible influencing factors or recent changes in influencing factors.
- General health including psychological factors.
- Current medication.
- Impact of constipation on quality of life.
- What has worked in the past?
- Physical examination – inspection, auscultation, palpation, percussion.

Pharmacological interventions to reduce constipation are shown in Table 44.2.

Procedure – Nursing Management

Ongoing care involves:

- Assessing effectiveness of any pharmacological intervention.
- Encouraging a fibre-rich diet.
- Encouraging an increased fluid intake.
- Encouraging exercise where possible.
- Discussing correct positioning for opening your bowels, providing a footstool if required (Figure 44.1).

Bowel Sounds

Traditionally, nurses have listened to bowel sounds as part of a wider abdominal assessment. The absence of bowel sounds, flatus and bowel movements, and the presence of nausea and vomiting, abdominal distension, bloating, or cramps may indicate impaired gut motility. However, the accuracy of assessing bowel sounds (Baid 2009) has been questioned and it has been considered of little benefit when assessing bowel obstruction (Bream et al. 2015). As there is no standardised approach, ensure that you are fully trained in this skill and refer to local policy when deciding whether to perform it in practice.

Procedure – Listening to Bowel Sounds

- The hands and diaphragm of the stethoscope should be warmed prior to touching the abdomen. This aims to prevent muscular contraction.
- Listen while moving systematically around all four quadrants of the abdomen (Figure 44.2).

NB: Excess pressure on the stethoscope diaphragm may stimulate peristalsis, so a light touch should be used.

Red Flags

- Rectal bleeding for six weeks or more.
- Change in bowel habit for six weeks or more.
- Palpable rectal mass.

References

Baid, H. (2009). A critical review of auscultating bowel sounds. *British Journal of Nursing* 18 (18): 1125–1129.

Bream, B.M., Rud, B., Kirkegarrd, T., and Norden, T. (2015). Accuracy of abdominal auscultation for bowel obstruction. *World Journal of Gastroenterology* 21 (34): 10018–10024.

45 Administration of suppositories and enemas

Figure 45.1   Correct position for rectal medication administration.

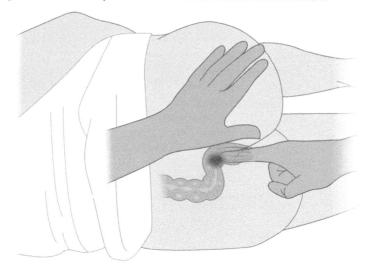

Figure 45.2   Suppositories.

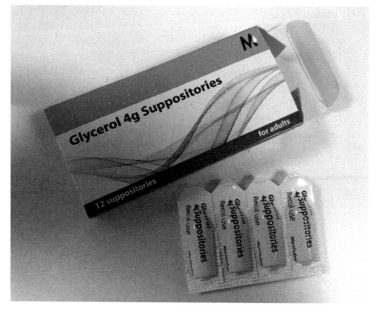

Figure 45.3   Enema.

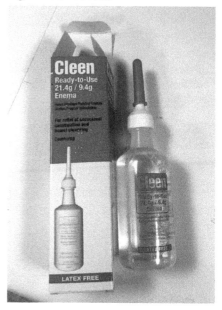

Clinical Nursing Skills at a Glance, First Edition. Edited by Sarah Curr and Carol Fordham-Clarke.
© 2022 John Wiley & Sons Ltd. Published 2022 by John Wiley & Sons Ltd.
Companion website: www.wiley.com/go/clinicalnursingskills

Background

Constipation can result from infrequent stools, less than three times per week, but can also be difficulty passing stools and a feeling of not fully emptying the bowel (NICE 2020). As such a full holistic assessment, using the Rome IV criteria (NICE 2020), will need to be undertaken and it may well be that medication is prescribed. Rectal administration of laxatives using enemas or suppositories may be appropriate in patients requiring rapid relief from constipation (Obokhare 2012). Enemas may also be used to evacuate the bowel prior to surgery. Always remember that these are medications and thus need to be prescribed and administered according to the correct principles.

Influencing Factors

- Gastrointestinal (GI) pathology, e.g. intestinal perforation, inflammatory bowel disease, rectal bleeding.
- Paralytic ileus.
- Colonic obstruction.
- Low platelet count.
- Perianal cancers (and radiotherapy).
- After GI/gynaecological surgery.
- Proctitis.

Professional Approach

- Introduce yourself to the client and gain informed consent.
- Accept the patient's right to refuse.
- Ensure privacy and keep the patient warm and covered where possible.
- Reassure the patient that the procedure can be stopped at any time.
- Take into consideration that the patient may find this procedure embarrassing.
- Ensure dignity by applying an incontinence sheet to the bed and having a commode or private toilet and the call bell nearby.
- Help the patient to lie on their left side with their knees drawn up to their chest (Lister, Hoftland, & Grafton, 2020) (Figure 45.1).
- Communicate sensitively throughout, explaining what you are doing.
- Always refer to the manufacturer's instructions when administering suppositories or enemas (Figures 45.2 & 45.3).

Equipment

- Appropriate suppository or enema.
- Lubricating gel as required.
- Continence support, i.e. disposable bed sheet.
- Commode or bed pan as required.

Procedure – Administering a Suppository

There is debate regarding the correct way to insert a suppository: blunt or rounded end first. Always read the manufacturer's instructions for definitive advice.

- Wash hands and put on gloves and apron.
- Lubricate the suppository as per manufacturer's instructions.
- Ask the patient to relax, lying on left side.

- Separate the patient's buttocks and advance the suppository 2–4 cm into the rectum.
- Clean excess lubricant from the perianal area and dry the area thoroughly.
- Ask the patient to retain the suppository according to manufacturer's instructions.
- Maintain patient hygiene.
- Dispose of waste according to infection control procedures and wash hands.
- Complete documentation.
- Assess effectiveness of intervention.

Procedure – Administering an Enema

- Warm the enema to room temperature by placing it in a jug of warm water according to manufacturer's instructions.
- Wash hands and put on gloves and apron.
- Express any excess air from the enema and lubricate the nozzle following manufacturer's instructions.
- Separate the buttocks and slowly introduce the nozzle into the anal canal.
- Ask the patient to relax.
- Advance the enema according to manufacturer's instructions.
- Fluid should be introduced by slowly rolling up the packaging from the base to the top to prevent backflow.
- Remove the nozzle gently and ask the patient to retain fluid according to manufacturer's instructions. Tilt the bed at 45° if appropriate.
- Clean any excess lubricant from the perianal area and dry the area thoroughly.
- Maintain patient hygiene.
- Dispose of waste according to infection control procedures and wash hands.
- Complete documentation.
- Assess effectiveness of intervention.

Red Flags

☛ Discontinue rectal administration if resistance is encountered.
☛ Rectal bleeding post-administration may indicate tissue damage.
☛ Phosphate enemas should be used with caution due to potential risks relating to phosphate absorption.

References

Cirocchi, R., Randolph, J., Panata., L., Verdelli, A.M., Mascagni, D., Mingoli, A., Zago, M., Chiarugi, M., Lancia, M., Fedeli, P., Davies, J., Occhionorelli, S. (2020) The tip of the iceberg of colorectal perforation from enema: a systematic review and meta-analysis. *Techniques in Coloproctology* 24 (2020), 1109–1119

Lister, S., Hoftland, J. & Grafton, H. (2020) The Royal Marsden Manual of Clinical Nursing Procedures, Professional Edition, 10th Edition. Oxford, Wiley-Blackwell

NICE (2020) Clinical Knowledge Summaries: Constipation. https://cks.nice.org.uk/topics/constipation/ (Accessed 11/08/2021)

Obokhare, I. (2012) Fecal impaction: a clinical cause for concern? *Clinics in Colon and Rectal Surgery* 25 (1), 53–58

46 Stoma care

Figure 46.1 Types of abdominal stoma.

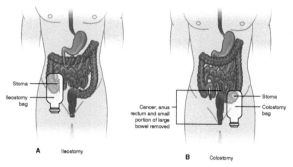

A   Ileostomy

Stoma
Ileostomy bag

B   Colostomy

Cancer, anus rectum and small portion of large bowel removed

Stoma
Colostomy bag

C   Urostomy/ileal conduit

Kidney
Ureter
Urostomy opening (Stoma)
Bowel used to carry urine (Ileal conduit)

Figure 46.4 Stoma powder.

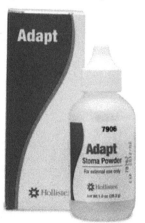

Adapt

7906

Adapt Stoma Powder
For external use only

Hollister

Figure 46.5 Skin protection barrier cream.

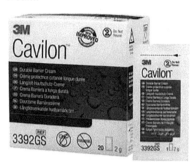

3M Cavilon
3392GS

Figure 46.2 Different types of stoma appliance.

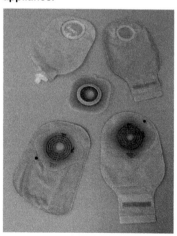

Figure 46.3 Fitting a colostomy flange.

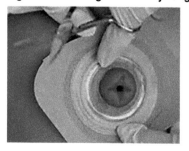

Table 46.1 Types of stoma.

Stoma/Location	Appearance
Colostomy • A section of the colon is resected. • Commonly, colostomies are formed on the left side of the abdomen • Output is soft, formed faeces and flatus	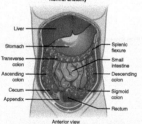 Stoma
Ileostomy • Part or all of the colon is resected and the stoma is formed from the ileum • Output is loose faecal matter and flatus • This stoma is raised to allow drainage of content, reducing excoriation of skin	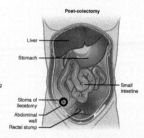 Complete colectomy with ileostomy
Urostomy or ileal conduit • The bladder is bypassed by inserting the ureters into a segment of ileum which is brought to the skin surface • Output is urine and a small amount of mucus	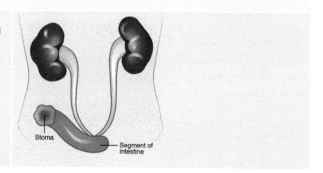

Clinical Nursing Skills at a Glance, First Edition. Edited by Sarah Curr and Carol Fordham-Clarke.
© 2022 John Wiley & Sons Ltd. Published 2022 by John Wiley & Sons Ltd.
Companion website: www.wiley.com/go/clinicalnursingskills

Background

A stoma is an opening made into a hollow organ primarily to allow drainage. Commonly stomas are formed due to cancer, inflammatory disorders or trauma. Stomas can be temporary or permanent and there are three abdominal types: ileostomy, colostomy, and urostomy/ileal conduit (Figure 46.1 and Table 46.1).

Influencing Factors

The type of stoma will influence the appliance used and the risk of skin conditions: e.g. ileostomy contents are potentially more corrosive.

Professional Approach

- Introduce yourself to the patient, explain the procedure, and obtain informed consent.
- Establish rapport and start building a therapeutic relationship.
- Ensure privacy and dignity during appliance changes.
- Be mindful that your client may be coming to terms with a change in body image related to stoma formation. Allow them time to express any concerns (Burch 2016).
- Where possible, encourage independence when managing a stoma, involving the patient in all aspects of stoma care, including assessment of the stoma and surrounding skin.
- Work within your own limitations as part of the multidisciplinary team, liaising with the stoma nurse specialist or surgical team as appropriate.

Equipment

- Ensure that you have the correct stoma appliance.
- Medical adhesive remover as required.
- Skin protective cream as appropriate.
- Soft cloths to clean and dry the area.
- Bowl for water.

Types of Appliances

Appliances come as either one piece with the adhesive flange attached to the bag, or as a two-piece, where the flange and bag are separate. There are also drainable bags available which allow frequent drainage without the need to change the bag on each emptying. Choice of appliance is dependent upon type of stoma and patient preference (Figure 46.2):

- A colostomy bag is usually a closed bag that is completely removed on each change.
- An ileostomy bag is usually a drainable bag.
- A urostomy bag is a drainable bag with a tap.

Procedure – Changing an Appliance

- Collect all necessary equipment.
- Ensure privacy for patient.
- Wash hands and put on gloves and apron.
- Protect the patient's clothing with an absorbent pad.
- Empty the bag if necessary.

- Gently remove the old appliance using one hand to support the skin and the other hand to peel the appliance away from the skin.
- Clean and dry the peri-stomal area using soft cloths.
- A mild, unperfumed soap can be used, but be aware this can dry the skin.
- Check the stoma and surrounding skin for:
  - Colour.
  - Bleeding.
  - Soreness or ulceration.
- Apply skin protection barrier as appropriate; this is particularly important with an ileostomy.
- Apply fresh appliance over stoma and hold in place for 30–60 seconds to help adhesion.
- Dispose of waste and perform hand hygiene in line with local policy.
- Document stoma assessment and appliance changes as per local policy.

Procedure – Managing Complications

- If there is discomfort on removing the old appliance, adhesive removal spray or wipes are available if required.
- Sore skin – ensure that the appliance flange is cut to the correct size; 1–2 mm larger than the stoma and the correct shape (Figure 46.3).
- Skin protection barrier creams, sprays, or wipes can be used on intact peri-stomal skin. Stoma powder can be applied to broken skin (Figures 46.4 and 46.5).
- A two-piece appliance will reduce the number of full appliance changes required, thus protecting the skin.
- Leaking appliance – ensure stoma is at the centre of flange opening and the flange has a flat, even base. Drain the appliance regularly. Follow the manufacturer's instructions on frequency of appliance change. Stoma seals, flange extensions, and belts are available to maximise adhesion.
- If there is any change in stoma appearance, contact medical team immediately.

Red Flags

- If there is an increase in stoma output, monitor for dehydration.
- If urostomy output smells offensive, screen for urinary tract infection.
- In the case of a prolapsed or retracted stoma, liaise with the stoma nurse specialist or surgical team.
- Dusky-coloured stomas indicate compromised perfusion requiring immediate escalation.

References

Burch, J. (2016). Exploring quality of life for stoma patients living in the community. *British Journal of Community Nursing* 21 (8): 378–382.

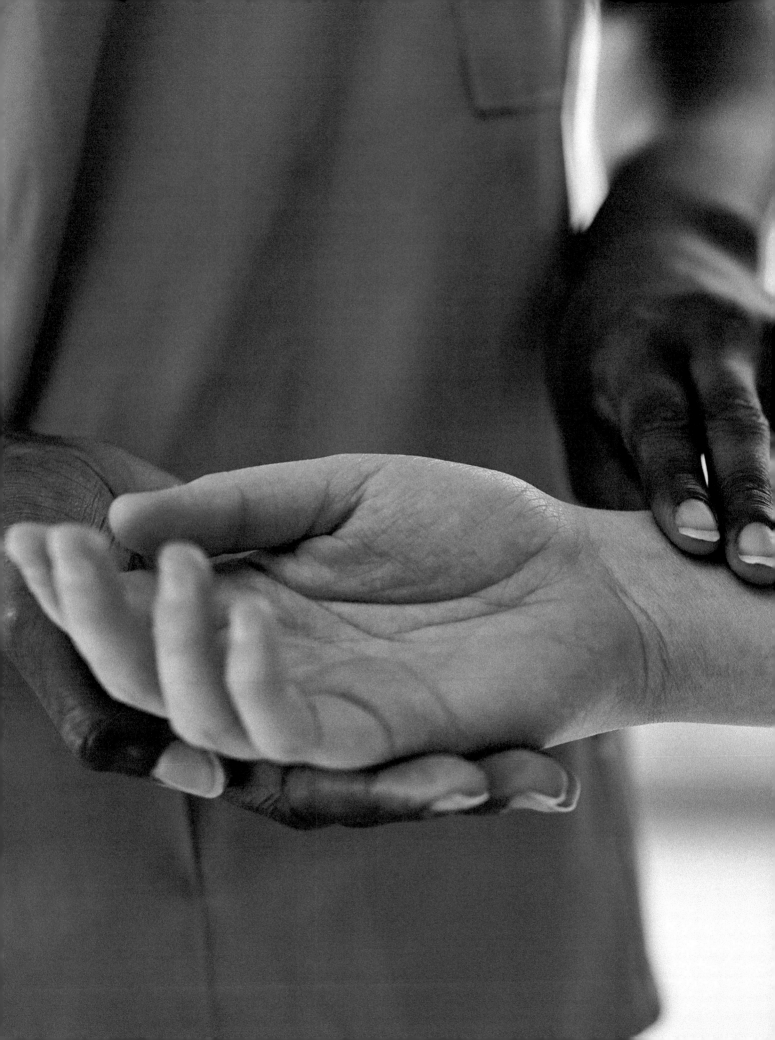

Genitourinary skills

Chapters

47 Urinalysis

Figure 47.1 Urinary system.

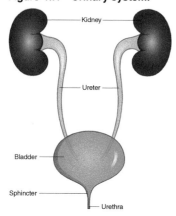

Kidney

Ureter

Bladder

Sphincter

Urethra

Figure 47.2 ANTT Catheter specimen of urine (CSU) from a port site.

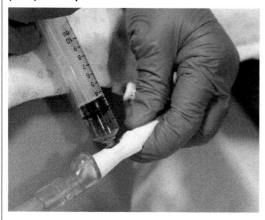

Figure 47.3 Reagent strip submersion.

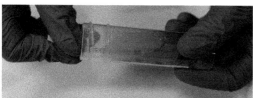

Figure 47.4 Reading reagent strip (hold horizontally).

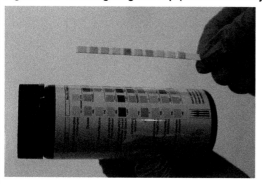

Table 47.1 Significance of urinalysis results.

Finding	Meaning
Colour	Brown or dark yellow could suggest bilirubin. Dark urine could suggest dehydration. Green could indicate infection, specifically pseudomonas. Bright red or red/brown suggests blood which could indicate kidney damage but menstruation should be ruled out
Clarity	Cloudiness could be pus as well as white blood cells thus indicating infection
Smell	A strong smell could be a result of food or drink consumed. A fishy, ammonia, or offensive smell is indicative of infection. A sweet smell could suggest ketones
Protein, proteinuria	Suggests a problem with kidney filtration in the glomerulus
Leucocytes, white blood cells, leucocyte esterase	Inflammation and/or infection in the body
Nitrites, from breakdown of nitrates	Usually indicative of a urinary tract infection; not all bacteria will convert nitrates to nitrites and these could be present if a suboptimal sampling technique has been performed
Blood, haematuria	This can be a sign of trauma or of infection such as cystitis or pyelonephritis. Larger amounts of blood can indicate kidney stones or some cancers
Specific gravity	The concentration of excreted molecules in the urine. An increase in specific gravity can be an indication of dehydration, whereas a decrease in specific gravity may suggest excessive fluid intake
Glucose, glycosuria	Associated with elevated blood glucose levels
pH	Normally between 4.5 and 8, but it is important to recognise that urine is often slightly acidic due to metabolic activity
Ketones, ketonuria	Waste product, when the body breaks down fat for energy; sometimes present in cases of dehydration, but can also be a sign of diabetic ketoacidosis
Bilirubin	Bilirubin is formed when red blood cells break down and this usually occurs in the liver. Bilirubin in the urine suggests that the liver is not working effectively

Figure 47.5 Documenting urinalysis results.

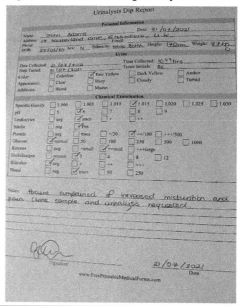

Clinical Nursing Skills at a Glance, First Edition. Edited by Sarah Curr and Carol Fordham-Clarke.
© 2022 John Wiley & Sons Ltd. Published 2022 by John Wiley & Sons Ltd.
Companion website: www.wiley.com/go/clinicalnursingskills

Background

- Urine is a waste product made by the kidneys and excreted by the body through the urethra (Figure 47.1).
- It is primarily made up of urea, chloride, and sodium, as well as potassium and creatinine.
- Other composites can also be excreted in urine, such as protein and hormones.
- Urinalysis is a fundamental clinical skill to screen for many health issues by ascertaining what is being excreted and how much of it.
- This can determine baseline data and can be used for comparisons for continuing care.
- Urinalysis can be undertaken on 24-hour collections, midstream urine (MSU) or catheter specimens of urine (CSU).

Influencing Factors

- Certain substances can affect urinalysis, e.g. asparagus through smell, beetroot through colour.
- Those receiving vitamin B, specifically thiamine, can have bright yellow urine, which could also indicate bilirubin, hence the importance of full patient history-taking.

Professional Approach

- Explain the procedure and why it is being performed to obtain informed consent.
- Provide clear instructions on how to provide the sample and ensure these are understood.
- Patients who are confused and/or incontinent will often require a urinalysis and time must be taken to explain why this is required.
- Those with a cognitive impairment may not be able to provide an uncontaminated sample and thus a fresh sample, with support as required, is recommended.
- Ensure that the sample is fresh, as long-standing samples will produce false-positives.
- Consider privacy and dignity and provide the patient with a secure area to leave the sample.
- Ensure that you are aware of what the results indicate (Table 47.1) to ensure that appropriate care and treatment are provided.

   NB: In certain circumstances, it may be in the patient's best interest to undertake intermittent catheterisation to obtain a sample.

Equipment

- Reagent strips.
- Sterile sample collection container.
- Sterile gauze.
- PPE (personal protective equipment) – single-use disposable gloves and apron.

Procedure

- In a mobile patient provide a clean receptacle, either a gallipot, jug, or a specimen bottle, to be used independently.
- In the immobile patient, a gallipot can be placed in a bedpan.
- In a catheterised patient a sample is not recommended for dipstick urinalysis (RCN 2019), but if a catheter associated urinary tract infection (CAUTI) is suspected a sample for microscopic cultures and sensitivity (MC&S) will be required. This must be taken from the catheter port site using an aseptic non-touch approach (ANTT) (Figure 47.2). Prior to inserting the syringe, the catheter drainage tube should be clamped, and the port cleaned with a 70% isopropyl alcohol solution (Loveday et al. 2014).
- Ask the patient to urinate into the clean receptacle and leave the sample in a pre-arranged area.
- Check reagent strips are intact and in date.
- Ensure your hands are washed or cleansed with alcohol hand rub and apply gloves and apron.
- Note the colour of the urine, i.e. dark brown, bright yellow, red (Yates 2016).
- Note the clarity of the sample (Martin and Martin 2019), i.e. clear, cloudy.
- Note the urine smell, i.e. fishy, offensive, sweet.
- Open the reagent strip container, remove one strip, and then close the container to avoid moisture causing the remaining strips to deteriorate.
- Dip the reagent strip into the urine, ensuring that all parts are covered in urine, then remove (Figure 47.3). A urine sample of 50 mL is usually sufficient to achieve this.
- Tap the reagent strip against the sample collection container to remove excess urine and then place on a paper towel to prevent contamination of the surface.
- Follow the reagent strip manufacturer's guidance regarding interpreting the results in the appropriate time-frame (usually one to three minutes) while holding the reagent strip horizontally,[1] adjacent to the reagent strip container (Figure 47.4).
- Read the results alongside the table on the container in good light to ensure accurate readings.
- Document findings (Figure 47.5) and escalate as appropriate.

Red Flags

- Protein can be an early sign of pre-eclampsia.
- Nitrites can be indicative of a UTI and, if left untreated, can cause pyelonephritis.
- Ketones associated with glucose either in the urine or through a blood glucose level can indicate diabetic ketoacidosis. This requires urgent intervention.

References

Loveday, H., Wilson, J.A., Pratt, R. et al. (2014). epic3: National Evidence-Based Guidelines for preventing healthcare-associated infections in NHS hospitals in England. *Journal of Hospital Infection* 86: S1–S70.
Martin, C. and Martin, H. (2019). Urinalysis using a test strip. *British Journal of Nursing* 28 (6): 336–340.
Royal College of Nursing (2019). *Catheter Care: RCN Guidance for Health Care Professionals*. London: Royal College of Nursing.
Yates, A. (2016). Urinalysis how to interpret results. *Nursing Times* 112 (2): 1–3.

[1] Holding the reagent strip horizontally prevents colours running together on the reagent strip. If this does occur, a new strip will be required.

48 # Continence assessment

Figure 48.1 Sphincter muscle controlling continence.

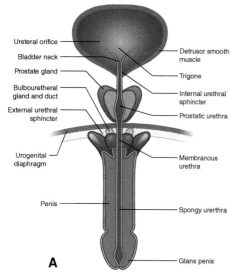

A

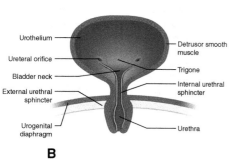

B

Figure 48.2 Female incontinence products.

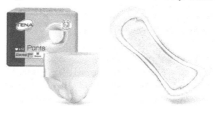

Figure 48.3 Male incontinence products.

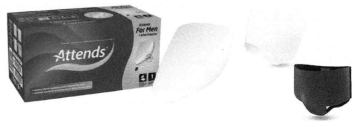

Figure 48.4 Incontinence bedding and chair covers.

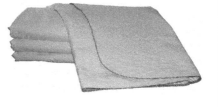
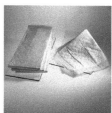

Table 48.1 Different types of incontinence.

Type of incontinence	Signs and symptoms
Urgency urinary incontinence	This type of incontinence occurs when a person feels the urge to go to the toilet but cannot control their bladder to get there in time. This can be caused by damage to the nerves that supply the bladder, but can also be a result of Multiple Sclerosis, Parkinson's disease, and Cerebrovascular Accident.
Stress urinary incontinence	This occurs when stress is placed on the pelvic floor, such as when laughing or coughing, and is commonly seen in women who are pregnant or who have had children.
Mixed urinary incontinence	This is a combination of stress and urgency urinary incontinence.
Functional urinary incontinence	Unlike the other types of incontinence, this type does not involve a problem with the urinary tract or pelvic floor. Functional incontinence occurs in people who may have a physical or mental impairment, such as arthritis or dementia, which inhibits them from getting to the bathroom in time.
Continuous urinary incontinence	This can happen when the bladder is full, but the person is unable to empty it, leading to leakage and dribbling. If a patient is unable to empty their bladder, this is referred to as retention of urine and can be very painful and potentially dangerous if left untreated. These patients will require a bladder scan to establish residual volume of urine prior to potential catheterisation. This type of scan is handheld and uses ultrasound technique to give an approximate amount of urine in millilitres. Prostate enlargement, constipation, and tumours are all causes of this type of incontinence.

Clinical Nursing Skills at a Glance, First Edition. Edited by Sarah Curr and Carol Fordham-Clarke.
© 2022 John Wiley & Sons Ltd. Published 2022 by John Wiley & Sons Ltd.
Companion website: www.wiley.com/go/clinicalnursingskills

Background

Normal bladder emptying involves sphincter muscles that maintain continence (Figure 48.1.) If these are not functioning effectively, urinary incontinence can result.

Urinary incontinence can be defined as "the complaint of any involuntary loss of urine" (D'Ancona et al. 2019, p. 4). This incontinence can affect both men and women, but it is thought that women are more affected due to damage sustained to the pelvic floor during pregnancy (Sangswang and Serisathien 2012). This means that how incontinence affects men can be overlooked (Esparza et al. 2018) and it is essential that a full holistic assessment is undertaken that considers each individual and their requirements.

It has also been recognised that episodes of incontinence appear to increase with age (Bardsley 2016), but it is not an inevitable part of ageing. It is currently estimated that 14 million people in the UK are affected by bladder problems (NHSE 2018) with at least three million of these being urinary (BAUS 2020).

Influencing Factors

Urinary incontinence can be a result of:

- Childbirth.
- Injuries during childbirth.
- Neurological disorders.
- Constipation.

Professional Approach

- Where possible have the conversation in a private environment in which the patient may feel more comfortable discussing this sensitive issue.
- Remember that the patient may not feel comfortable discussing their urinary incontinence with you, and offer the opportunity to discuss with a colleague if you notice discomfort.
- Reassure the patient that this is common and there are many effective management strategies.

Procedure

The most common types of urinary incontinence are:

- Urgency urinary incontinence.
- Stress urinary incontinence.
- Mixed urinary incontinence.
- Functional urinary incontinence.
- Continuous urinary incontinence (Table 48.1).

Although there is no standardised tool for assessing urinary incontinence, the questions below will help to ascertain which type of urinary incontinence the patient may be experiencing:

- How often is it happening?
- How much urine are you leaking?
- What makes it worse?
- What makes it better?
- Does it stop you from doing anything?
- What products/techniques do you currently use to control it?

Asking broad questions provides an opportunity for the patient to explain the effect that urinary incontinence is having on their life. It also enables you to determine the type of continence by considering the questions to ask. Continence nurse specialists and urology specialists can be a useful resource when undertaking a more detailed assessment.

- Introduce yourself to the patient and explain that you are undertaking a urinary incontinence assessment and what that entails.
- Close the door or curtain to provide as much privacy as possible.

- Ask the questions detailed above to ascertain what type of urinary incontinence might be present.
- Advise that a urinalysis will need to be undertaken and the process for this (Chapter 47).
- If the patient is complaining of voiding problems, advise that a bladder scan, to ascertain residual urine, is likely.

Managing Urinary Incontinence

Offer patients the variety of urinary incontinence products available within your organisation. These may include:

- Female incontinence products (Figure 48.2).
- Male incontinence products (Figure 48.3).
- Bedding and chair covers (Figure 48.4).

Remember that there will be individual preference and some people will prefer the security of a larger pad, while others may be more focused on comfort (Buckley 2017). Similarly, men may choose to use women's products and vice versa. For women, there is an option to receive pelvic floor strengthening exercises from a physiotherapist during and/or after pregnancy if they wish (NICE 2019).

Undertaking a thorough assessment and obtaining a clear management plan are essential to ensure that patients are comfortable and can undertake their activities of daily living. For some people, surgery may be required (NICE 2019) but this may not always be appropriate or possible and as such patients who may be more dependent must have good continence management to maintain personal dignity and skin integrity, and to prevent infection and sustain a good quality of life.

Red Flags

- ☛ New incontinence following back injuries should be treated as an emergency as this can be an indication of nerve damage or cauda equina syndrome.
- ☛ Dribbling small amounts of urine frequently can be a sign of urinary retention, especially in men.

References

Bardsley, A. (2016). An overview of urinary incontinence. *The British Journal of Nursing* 25 (18): 537–545.

British Association of Urological Surgeons (BAUS) (2020) *I think I Might Have . . . Incontinence of Urine.* https://www.baus.org.uk/patients/conditions/5/incontinence_of_urine (accessed 14 November 2020).

Buckley, B.S. (2017). User perspectives, preferences and priorities relating to products for managing bladder and bowel dysfunctions. *Journal of Engineering in Medicine* 233 (1): 7–18.

D'Ancona, C.D., Haylen, B.T., Oelke, M. et al. (2019). An International Continence Society (ICS) report on the terminology for adult male lower urinary tract and pelvic floor Symptoms and dysfunction. *Neurourology and Urodynamics* 38 (2): 433–477.

Esparza, A.O., Tomás, M.A.C., and Pina-Roche, F. (2018). Experiences of women and men living with urinary incontinence: a phenomenological study. *Applied Nursing Research* 40: 68–75.

National Health Service England (2018). *Excellence in Continence Care: Practical Guide for Commissioners, and Leaders in Health and Social Care.* Leeds: NHS England.

National Institute of Health and Care Excellence (2019). *NG123: Urinary Incontinence and Pelvic Organ Prolapse in Women: Management.* London: National Institute of Health and Care Excellence.

Sangswang, B. and Serisathien, Y. (2012). Effect of pelvic floor muscle exercise programme on stress urinary incontinence among pregnant women. *Journal of Advanced Nursing* 68 (9): 1997–2007.

49 Urinary catheterisation

Figure 49.1 Catheter balloon.

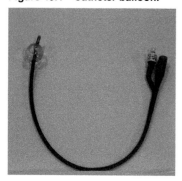

Figure 49.4 Urometer and catheter bags.

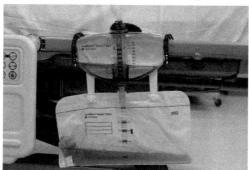

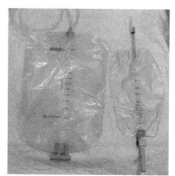

Figure 49.2 Male and female catheters.

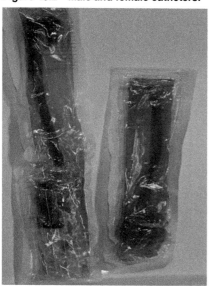

Figure 49.5 Tear along the perforated edge.

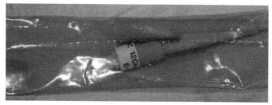

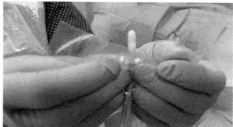

Figure 49.3 Catheterisation equipment.

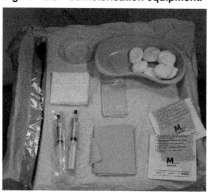

Figure 49.6 Male catheterisation.

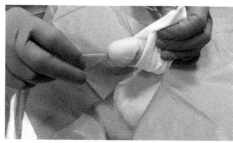

Figure 49.7 Inflate the balloon.

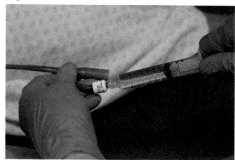

Clinical Nursing Skills at a Glance, First Edition. Edited by Sarah Curr and Carol Fordham-Clarke.
© 2022 John Wiley & Sons Ltd. Published 2022 by John Wiley & Sons Ltd.
Companion website: www.wiley.com/go/clinicalnursingskills

Background

Urinary catheters are small tubes inserted into the bladder to drain urine. They are held in place by a small, inflatable balloon (Figure 49.1) and may be inserted for:

- Chronic incontinence – i.e. following injury to the nervous system.
- Urinary retention – often a result of benign prostatic hyperplasia in men.
- Post-surgery – either to monitor urine output or to rest the bladder.
- Critically unwell patients – for fluid balance.
- Irrigation – for haematuria or clot retention.

This section will discuss urethral catheters (male and female), insertion, and approach. Suprapubic catheter placement is a specialist skill and requires further training.

NB: Urinary catheters are not routinely inserted for continence management. Catheter insertion in this instance will need to be a multidisciplinary team decision that must be discussed with the patient, with the risks of having an indwelling catheter considered.

Influencing Factors

- Some patients may be unable to provide informed consent. In such circumstances, capacity and best interests will need to be considered.
- An enlarged prostrate can result in it being difficult to pass the catheter; in such instances referral to a urology specialist is recommended.

Professional Approach

- Full use of communication skills is required to help the patient feel comfortable.
- Cover the patient when they no longer need to be exposed – being professional throughout will help to maintain privacy and dignity.
- For patient comfort and safety, select the most appropriate catheter, the one with the smallest gauge that will allow urinary flow (Loveday et al. 2014).

Catheter Sizes

- Catheters have different widths and are measured in Charrières (ch) or French gauge (FG).
- Generally use a 12ch or 14ch for women and a 14ch or 16ch for men. A larger catheter may be used for irrigation purposes or post-surgery.
- Catheters come in two lengths – standard and female (Figure 49.2). Female catheters should not be inserted into men. They are not long enough to reach the bladder, and if the balloon were inflated it could damage the urethra.
- Catheters are also available for short-term (up to 4 weeks) or longer-term use (usually up to 12 weeks) that are made of silicone to reduce the infection risk.

Equipment

Before you start you will need the following (Figure 49.3):

- A clean dressing trolley.
- A catheter or standard dressing pack.
- A catheter and prefilled syringe.
- 10 mL syringe and sterile water if required.
- Two pairs of sterile gloves.
- Local anaesthetic (LA) lubricant.
- Cleaning agent – 0.9% sodium chloride.
- A catheter bag or urometer (Figure 49.4a,b).
- A clinical waste bag.

Procedure

- Explain why the catheter is being inserted, obtain informed consent, explain the procedure, and highlight that it should not be painful.
- Wash hands and put on personal protective equipment (PPE).
- Prepare your sterile field.

NB: Although urethral catheters are not being inserted into an area that can be sterilised, it is still important to maintain aseptic non-touch technique to reduce the risk of cross-contamination.

- Check that all equipment is intact and in date.
- Open LA lubricant and catheter onto sterile field.
- Empty 0.9% sodium chloride into the gallipot.
- Ensure that that you have good access to the urethral opening. Ask women to bend their knees up and relax them out to the side. For men, keep legs straight and retract the foreskin.
- Decontaminate hands and apply sterile gloves.
- Use a sterile drape either over the top of the patient, with the hole exposing the urethral opening, or under the patient as an extension of the sterile field.
- Clean the urethral opening using 0.9% sodium chloride, or other solution if prescribed, until visibly clean. Ensure that wiping occurs away from the urethra by wiping down in women or in a spiral motion for men.
- Apply lubricant into the urethral opening. For men, the penis should be held perpendicular using a piece of sterile gauze to prevent contamination of gloves. Use 6 mL for women and 11 mL for men and leave for three to five minutes (Lister et al. 2020) to allow the anaesthetic to work.
- Change the sterile gloves.
- Tear the catheter along the perforation, at the tip, to expose the end (Figure 49.5). Insert the catheter.
- In men, insert the initial 10 cm into the penis held upright, using sterile gauze (Figure 49.6); when resistance is felt, lower penis and continue.
- Advance the catheter until urine appears in the outer plastic cover.
- Remove the plastic cover and rest the end of the catheter in the sterile dish.
- Inflate the balloon using the pre-filled syringe or 10 mL sterile water determined by the manufacturer's guidance (Figure 49.7).
- Attach the catheter bag/urometer using a non-touch technique.
- With male catheterisation ensure that the foreskin is put back into place.
- Leave your patient comfortable and dispose of your waste in the clinical waste bin. Wipe any LA displaced by the catheter.
- Document the insertion in the patient's notes using the appropriate documentation, including size, date, and amount of sterile water used to inflate balloon.

Red Flags

- Anuria, oliguria, and polyurea require investigation.
- Unexpected haematuria should be reported immediately as it is a potential sign of damage to the urethra.
- Not replacing the foreskin can cause paraphimosis and thus irreversible damage.
- Hypospadias, while normal for some men, can create a false passage. These patients may need to be catheterised by a specialist.
- Do not force a catheter that will not advance as the patient may have a urethral stricture. In men, this is commonly caused by the prostate and may need a specialist assessment.

References

Lister, S., Hofland, J., and Grafton, H. (2020). *The Royal Marsden Manual of Clinical Nursing Procedures*, 10e. Professional Edition. Chichester: Wiley Blackwell.

Loveday, H., Wilson, J.A., Pratt, R. et al. (2014). epic3: National Evidence-Based Guidelines for preventing healthcare-associated infections in NHS hospitals in England. *Journal of Hospital Infection* 86: S1–S70.

50 Catheter care

Figure 50.1   StatLock stabilisation device.

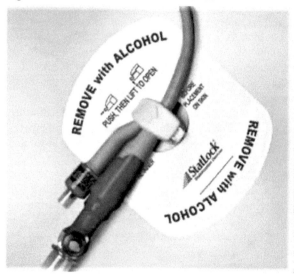

Figure 50.2   Adjust tap for free drainage.

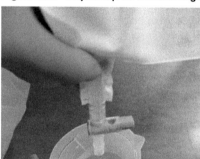

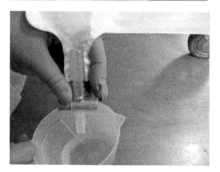

Figure 50.3   Catheter bag on a stand.

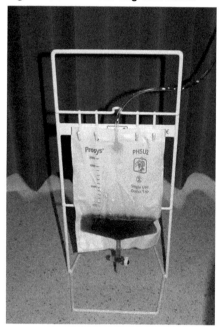

Figure 50.4   Open (a) and closed (b) catheter clamp.

(a)

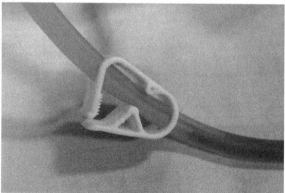

(b)

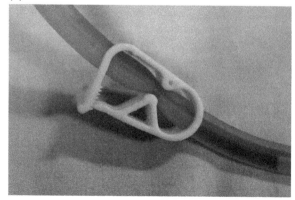

Background

It is recognised that there is an increased likelihood of finding bacteria the longer a catheter stays in place and that after one month of having an indwelling catheter, all individuals living with a catheter will have evidence of bacteriuria (NICE 2018). As such, catheter care is of utmost importance. Although this must be provided daily in the in hospital setting, it is imperative that the person living with a catheter is shown how to provide self-care and provided with information on the catheter. This usually takes the form of a catheter passport (RCN 2019).

This section will provide details on how to provide catheter cleansing, and how to empty and change a catheter bag. Further information on other activities, such as intercourse, and troubleshooting can be found in the catheter passport (NHSE 2020).

Influencing Factors

- Some patients may find it difficult or may be unable to perform catheter care independently. Ensuring that the necessary support is provided is fundamental prior to discharge from the clinical setting. This may involve providing daily support for catheter care.
- Catheter care will be required daily for both suprapubic and urethral catheters. Urethral catheters will also require catheter care after going to the toilet and opening bowels (Loveday et al. 2014).
- It is recommended that a catheter bag is emptied:
  - once it is three-quarters full to prevent pulling of the catheter.
  - when the bladder feels full.
  - prior to opening the bowels.
- The catheter bag should be changed every seven days or in accordance with manufacturer's instructions.

Professional Approach

- Consider privacy and dignity by ensuring that you explain exactly what is being undertaken.
- Provide the patient with the opportunity for a chaperone or for another member of staff to undertake the procedure.
- To avoid risk of catheter pull, ensure that a stabilising device is used, e.g. a StatLock (Figure 50.1).

Equipment – Catheter Care

Before you start you will need the following:

- Disposable gloves and single-use apron.
- Non-perfumed soap and water.
- Disposable patient cleansing wipes.

Procedure – Catheter Care

- Communicate the rationale for catheter care and explain what care needs to be provided.
- Ensure that written instructions are given (usually in the form of a catheter passport).
- Ensure that the curtain or door is closed.
- Wash hands and put on personal protective equipment (PPE).
- Ensure patient comfort and expose the genitalia only.
- Observe the meatus for any signs of infection or irritation.
- For women, cleanse the meatus ensuring that you wash front to back.
- For men use a spiral motion when cleansing. If the patient has a foreskin, ensure that you cleanse under the retracted foreskin before it is replaced.
- For suprapubic catheters, look for leakage at site.
- Wash the catheter tubing away from the body.
- Use disposable wipes to dry the area after cleansing in accordance with local policy.
- Document care provided.

Equipment – Emptying a Catheter Bag

- Disposable gloves and single use apron.
- Appropriate receptacle.

Procedure – Emptying a Catheter Bag

- Explain that you are emptying the catheter bag and why this is being performed.
- Note the colour of the urine.
- Assess the system, ensuring that it remains closed.
- Ensure that the receptable is placed directly under the bag drainage tap.
- Adjust tap to ensure free drainage (Figure 50.2).
- Close tap once drainage is complete.
- Ensure that the bag is below the level of the bladder to avoid reflux and remains a closed system (RCN 2019).
- If the catheter bag is on a stand, ensure that neither the bag nor the tap touches the floor (Figure 50.3) to avoid contamination.
- Document fluid balance if required.

Equipment – Changing a Catheter Bag

- Disposable gloves and single-use apron.
- Appropriate sterile catheter bag.
- Securing equipment.
- Clinical waste bag.

Procedure – Changing a Catheter Bag

- Empty the catheter bag using the above technique.
- Clamp the catheter tubing to prevent leakage (Figure 50.4).
- Remove leg bands or other securing equipment.
- Remove the top from the new catheter bag.
- Remove the attached catheter bag using a twisting motion and place in a clinical waste bag.
- Attach the new bag using a twisting motion, ensuring that a non-touch technique is used.
- Secure bag using leg bands or other equipment.
- Document actions taken.

NB: If using a night bag this should be attached to the leg bag tap ensuring that the tap is in the open drainage position. It is recommended that single-use night bags are used (RCN 2019).

Red Flags

- No urine drainage in the catheter bag over several hours could suggest blockage and the patient needs to be assessed immediately by a trained professional.
- Not replacing the foreskin can cause paraphimosis and thus irreversible damage.
- Never reuse or wash drainage bags.
- Never reconnect used night bags.

References

Loveday, H., Wilson, J.A., Pratt, R. et al. (2014). epic3: National Evidence-Based Guidelines for preventing healthcare-associated infections in NHS hospitals in England. *Journal of Hospital Infection* 86: S1–S70.

National Health Service England (NHSE) (2020) *My Urinary Catheter Passport*. https://www.england.nhs.uk/wp-content/uploads/2020/08/Catheter_passport_v7.pdf (accessed 14 August 2020).

National Institute of Health and Care Excellence (2018). *NG113: Urinary Tract Infection (Catheter Associated): Antimicrobial Prescribing*. London: National Institute of Health and Care Excellence.

Royal College of Nursing (2019). *Catheter Care: RCN Guidance for Health Care Professionals*. London: Royal College of Nursing.

51 Catheter removal

Figure 51.1 Intermittent catheters: male and female.

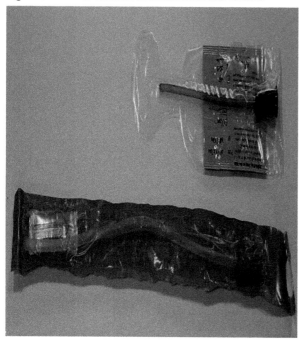

Figure 51.2 Suprapubic catheter placement. *Source: Redrawn from Pinder et al. (2015).*

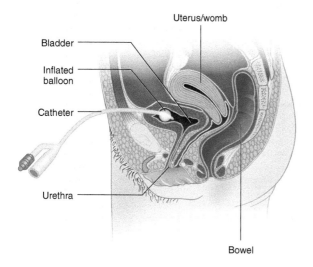

- Uterus/womb
- Bladder
- Inflated balloon
- Catheter
- Urethra
- Bowel

Figure 51.3 Drain balloon.

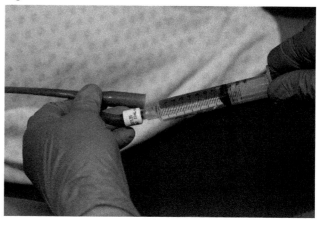

Table 51.1 Urinary retention: signs and symptoms.*

Urinary frequency

Urinary urgency

Straining to pass urine

Swelling of lower abdomen

Pain in lower abdomen

Flow that is weak with small amounts passed

* All these signs and symptoms require you to call a healthcare professional, usually the number provided in your catheter passport.

Background

As it is recognised that any indwelling device increases the risk of infection (Loveday et al. 2014) and that an indwelling catheter will develop bacteriuria within one month of insertion (NICE 2017), catheter removal is of paramount importance. Once the reason for catheterisation has resolved, a trial without catheter (TWOC) will be performed.

Although timely catheter removal is recommended once the need for a catheter has resolved (NICE 2017) there are some instances where the person may be unable to void without assistance, such as when there has been trauma affecting the nerves of the bladder, and while intermittent self-catheterisation is considered the gold standard (Pinder et al. 2015) (Figure 51.1) this may not always be possible. In these circumstances, a suprapubic catheter (Figure 51.2) or urethral catheter will be considered, and these indwelling devices will need to be maintained and changed.

Urethral catheter removal and re-insertion will also occur when the reason for insertion has not yet been remedied and the patient requires a catheter change. This change could be from a short-term catheter (up to three weeks) to a long-term catheter (12 weeks) on discharge from hospital or the change of a long-term catheter in the community. As such, this section will outline the procedure for removal of a catheter when there is a TWOC as well as when changing a catheter.

Influencing Factors

Care must be undertaken, and referral to specialist urology services considered, when removing a catheter in incidences when there:

- Are large uterine fibroids.
- Has been previous failed TWOCs.
- Has been surgery for stress incontinence.
- Is a large urogenital prolapse (RCN 2019).

TWOC time will depend upon the patient and can be:

- Late daytime, overnight, with review the next morning.
- At night for those with nocturnal polyuria.
- Early time for convenience (RCN 2019).

Professional Approach

- Consider privacy and dignity by ensuring that you explain exactly what is being undertaken.
- Provide the patient with the opportunity for a chaperone or for another member of staff to undertake the procedure.
- Consider whether the reason for catheter placement has been addressed.
- Check if the patient has benign prostatic hyperplasia – if so, alpha blockers may be prescribed prior to catheter removal (Fisher et al. 2014).

Equipment

Before you start you will need the following:

- Disposable gloves and single-use apron.
- Receptacle for catheter.
- 10 mL syringe.

Procedure

- Explain why the catheter is being removed and what the procedure involves in order to obtain informed consent.
- Encourage the patient to wash or shower before the procedure, if support is required provide this.
- Check the patient's notes to ascertain amount of sterile water inserted to fill the balloon.
- Ask the patient to rest in the supine position; assist as required.
- Decontaminate hands and put on gloves and apron.
- Place absorbent pad underneath the patient.
- Ensure that the catheter bag or urometer is empty.
- Remove all catheter support devices, i.e. StatLock, leg bands.
- Attach the syringe and allow the solution to drain out of the balloon into the syringe (Figure 51.3); do not pull on the syringe. Make a note of the solution amount in mL and dispose in the clinical waste.
- Advise the patient that you will now be removing the catheter and that, although there may be some discomfort, it should not be painful and to notify you if it is.
- Remove the catheter using continuous traction.
- Once removed, check for encrustation (Yates 2017).
- If inserting a new catheter, follow the procedure steps outlined in Chapter 49.
- Document actions, including water remaining in balloon, any encrustation, as well as date and time.
- With catheter removal without re-insertion (TWOC) encourage the patient to drink 1–2 L during the day.
- Advise patient of symptoms of urinary retention and what steps to take (Table 51.1).
- Advise an appointment time to review the success of TWOC.
- If in the in-patient setting, advise patient to alert you when they next need to void.

Red Flags

- ☛ Anuria and/or abnormal pain with a palpable bladder are indicative of acute urinary retention, a medical emergency that requires immediate treatment.
- ☛ Stop catheter removal if pain or excess bleeding is reported and if the patient requests you to stop.

References

Fisher, E., Subramonian, K. & Omar, M.I. (2014) The role of alpha blockers prior to removal of urethral catheter for acute urinary retention in men. Cochrane Database of Systematic Reviews. https://www.cochranelibrary.com/cdsr/doi/10.1002/14651858.CD006744.pub3/full (accessed 14 June 2021)

Loveday, H., Wilson, J.A., Pratt, R. et al. (2014). epic3: National Evidence-Based Guidelines for preventing healthcare-associated infections in NHS hospitals in England. *Journal of Hospital Infection* 86: S1–S70.

National Institute of Health and Care Excellence (2017). *[CG139]. Healthcare-associated Infections: Prevention and Control in Primary and Community Care*. London: National Institute of Health and Care Excellence.

Pinder, B., Lloyd, A.J., Nafee, B. et al. (2015). Patient preferences and willingness to pay for innovations in intermittent self-catheters. *Patient Preference and Adherence* 2015, 9: 381–388.

Royal College of Nursing (2019). *Catheter Care: RCN Guidance for Health Care Professionals*. London: Royal College of Nursing.

Yates, A. (2017). Urinary catheters 6: removing an indwelling catheter. *Nursing Times* 113 (6): 33–35.

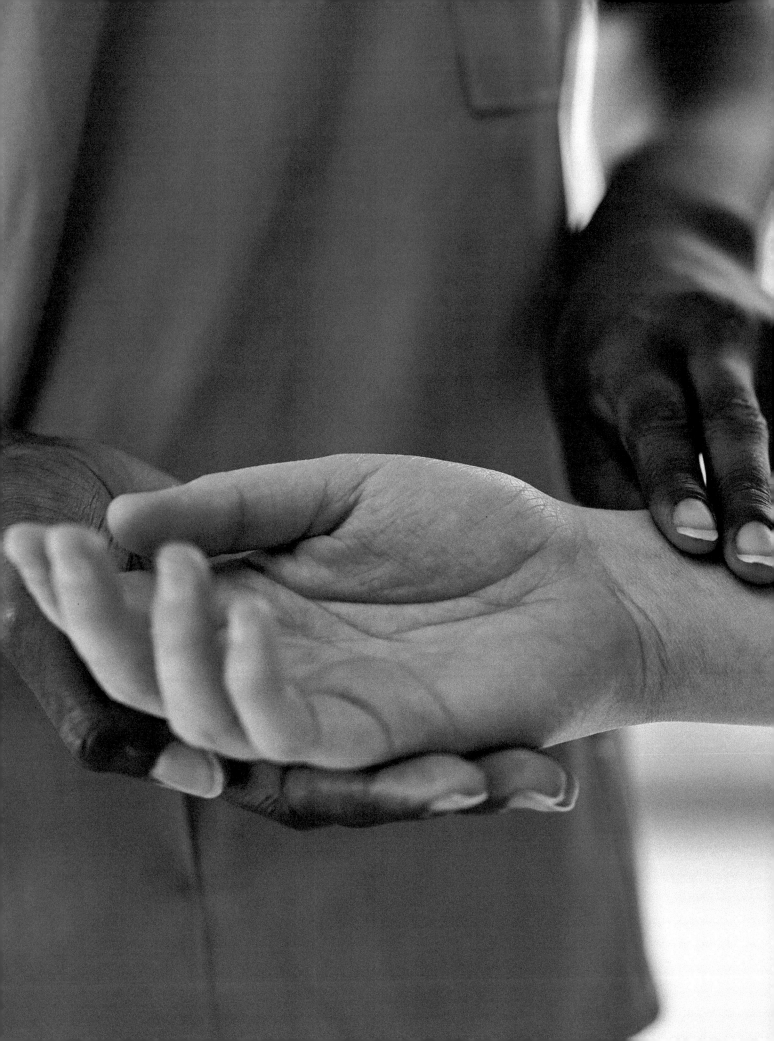

Musculoskeletal skills

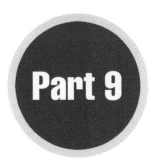

Chapters

52 Assessing tone and ability to mobilise

Figure 52.1 Muscle weakness/atrophy.

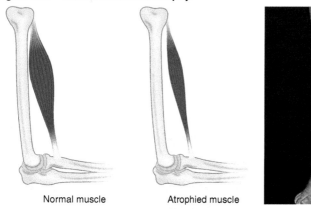

Normal muscle   Atrophied muscle

Figure 52.2 Postural malalignment.

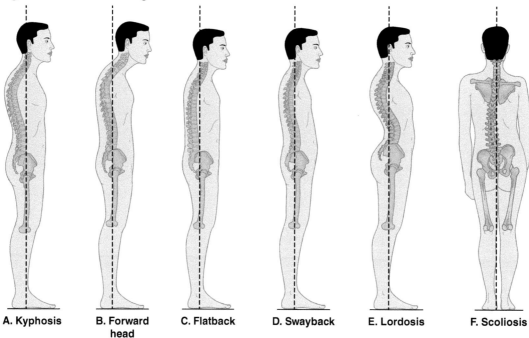

A. Kyphosis   B. Forward head   C. Flatback   D. Swayback   E. Lordosis   F. Scoliosis

Table 52.1 Timed Get Up and Go (TUG) test.

The following is timed:
* Patient stands up from a sitting position
* Walks 3 m (cane or walker may be used)
* Turns around, walks back to chair
* Sits down.

Patients showing unsteadiness or taking longer than 10 seconds require further assessment (Turner 2014).

Source: Based on Turner (2014).

Background

The act of movement is informed by the motor cortex in the brain but also involves bone, muscle and joint function (Marieb and Hoehn 2018). As brain, muscle, and bone health can be impacted upon by many acute and chronic conditions, the healthcare professional will need to assess mobility daily as part of care planning. This assessment of mobility will consider neurological function (Chapters 17 and 18) but also gait, core stability, bone strength and deformity, as well as muscle tone, strength and power. While much of this will be performed by a physiotherapist, due to their extensive and specialist training in this area (Porter 2013), there are some aspects that can be performed by other healthcare professionals when assessing capacity to mobilise. These are highlighted below.

Influencing Factors

There are multiple chronic and acute disorders that can affect mobility. Examples of these are:

- Neuromuscular disorders.
- Musculoskeletal conditions – acute or chronic.
- Arthritis – either osteoarthritis or rheumatoid arthritis.
- Cardiovascular conditions, i.e. heart failure, peripheral artery disease.
- Diabetes – specifically with neuropathy.
- Post-Cerebrovascular Accident.
- Mental health conditions.
- Chronic pain.

Professional Approach

When assessing the patient's mobility, the healthcare professional must recognise that this can change daily and will depend on the patients, what activities they undertook the day before, as well as treatments and analgesics being provided. As such, the patient should be assessed on every interaction, informed consent obtained, and the curtain or door closed as appropriate.

Procedure – History-taking

When assessing mobility, it is essential to:

- Listen – by obtaining an accurate history of usual mobility pattern, i.e. do they usually require a walking aid? Can they manage stairs? This ensures that safe and realistic goals are set.
- Listen – to ascertain if there is a history of any falls and the circumstances in which they occurred. This should be clearly documented.
- Perform – A psychological assessment, if competent, to establish the patient's motivation and if they are likely to experience anxiety when mobilising. This could impact on their ability to mobilise, and thus potentially make mobility unsafe.

NB: If, for any reason, the patient cannot provide an accurate history of mobility issues, a further history should be obtained from a current carer or next of kin/significant other.

Procedure – Preparing to Mobilise

- Prior to mobilisation, offer analgesia and allow adequate time for affect. Next perform a risk assessment, which involves:
  - Considering the patient's current physical health.
  - Considering any pre-existing conditions that may cause complications (see "Influencing Factors").
  - Recognising their ability to comply and follow instructions.
  - Considering any venous or arterial access devices, drips, or drains that might pose a risk.
  - Considering the patient's footwear; it should be sturdy and non-slip.
  - Considering the environment, ensuring that there is enough space and it is free of obstacles.

Procedure – Assessing Tone

Assessing tone establishes how much strength a patient has in their limbs and whether they will be able to support their own weight. The simplest way of doing this is to encourage the patient to move themselves in the bed or chair and look for:

- Asymmetry.
- Muscle wasting/atrophy (Figure 52.1).
- Weakness.
- Swelling.
- Bruising.
- Localised swelling.
- Redness.
- Deformity.

NB: If the patient is not able to move independently, it may be necessary to consider using a hoist rather than encouraging any weight-bearing activities.

Procedure – Assessing Muscle Strength

Muscle weakness may be reported when there is fatigue, slow reaction time or issues with gait (Penner and Paul 2017). As such a full history must be taken to assess the patient's primary complaint. If muscle strength needs to be assessed, each limb needs to be tested for weakness (Soames and Palastange 2018). Assessing passive and active movements, movement to resistance, and range of movement needs to be undertaken by a fully trained and competent individual. Basic limb strength assessment is discussed in Chapter 18.

Procedure – Assessing Gait and Power

Once the patient is standing it is possible to observe posture and look for any malalignment (Figure 52.2). If there is any cause for concern, the assessment should be discussed and a specialist assessment requested from a physiotherapist.

Once the patient is standing mobility, can be assessed by asking them to take a few steps. When the patient is walking, they should be observed for posture, gait and power.[1] Aim for a short distance if there has not been any recent mobilisation, and always put the safety of the patient first.

Frailty

Walking slow may suggest frailty in an older person. This can be assessed using the TUG test (see Table 52.1).

Red Flags

☛ If vascular or neurological compromise is suspected, do not mobilise.
☛ If there is excessive pain on mobilisation, stop immediately.

References

Marieb, E.N. and Hoehn, K. (2018). *Human Anatomy & Physiology*, 11e. Pearson: Harlow.
Penner, I.-K. and Paul, F. (2017). Fatigue as a symptom or comorbidity of neurological diseases. *Nature Reviews Neurology* 13 (2017): 662–675.
Porter, S. (2013). *Tidy's Physiotherapy*, 15e. Edinburgh: Churchill Livingstone.
Soames, R. and Palastange, N. (2018). *Anatomy and Human Movement Structure and Function*. Edinburgh: Churchill Livingstone.
Turner G (2014) Recognising frailty. https://www.bgs.org.uk/resources/recognising-frailty (accessed 24 May 2021).

---

1 Power is considered the work done versus the time taken (Soames and Palastange 2018) and this will give you an insight into physical well-being and endurance.

53 Venous thromboembolism assessment and risk reduction

Table 53.1 Venous thromboembolism (VTE) risk assessment.

DH (2018) guidelines state that a VTE risk assessment should include assessment of the following.

* Level of mobility:

  Normal state of mobility

  Any expected ongoing reduced mobility due to treatment

* Patient-related factors for thrombosis risk, including:

  Active cancer or cancer treatment

  Age >60 years

  Dehydration

  Known thrombophilia

  Body mass index >30 kg/m²

  Significant medical comorbidity, e.g. heart disease

  First-degree relative with history of VTE

  Hormone replacement therapy

  Contraceptive therapy

  Varicose veins with phlebitis

  Pregnancy

* Procedural-related risk factors, including:

  Reduced mobility >3 days

  Hip or knee replacement

  Hip fracture

  Anaesthetic time >90 minutes

  Critical care admission

  Surgery with significant reduction in mobility

* Assessment of patient related bleeding risk including:

  Active bleeding

  Acquired or inherited bleeding disorder

  Anticoagulant use

  Acute stroke

  Thrombocytopaenia

  Uncontrolled systolic hypertension

* Procedural-related bleeding risk including:

  Neurosurgery, spinal surgery, or eye surgery

Lumbar puncture or epidural anaesthesia expected within the next 12 hours or within the previous 4 hours

Source: Based on Department of Health (2018).

Table 53.2 Risk factors for venous thromboembolism (VTE).

Patient-related	Disease- or procedure-related
Age > 40 years	Heart failure
Immobility	Inflammatory bowel disease
Hormone replacement therapy	Malignancy
Contraceptive therapy	Nephrotic syndrome
Homocysteinaemia	Paralysis of lower limb(s)
Phospholipid antibody or lupus	Paraproteinaemia
Anticoagulant	Polycythaemia
Pregnancy	Recent myocardial infarction
Previous history of deep vein thrombosis or pulmonary embolism	Respiratory failure
Activated protein C resistance	Severe infection
Obesity	Trauma or surgery, especially of pelvis, hip, and lower limb
Smoking	Central venous catheterisation
Thrombophilias	
Varicose veins	

Clinical Nursing Skills at a Glance, First Edition. Edited by Sarah Curr and Carol Fordham-Clarke.
© 2022 John Wiley & Sons Ltd. Published 2022 by John Wiley & Sons Ltd.
Companion website: www.wiley.com/go/clinicalnursingskills

Background

Each year thousands of people die from hospital-acquired venous thromboembolism (VTE); the number of deaths was 11 696 in 2018–2019 (NHS Digital 2020) and as this is a highly preventable cause of death it needs to be addressed. VTE may occur both during admission or within 90 days of discharge, occurring most commonly in the deep veins of the legs or pelvis (NHS Digital 2020). A deep vein thrombosis (DVT) may cause pain and swelling in the leg but may also be asymptomatic (NICE 2018).

Thrombus dislodgement can cause a pulmonary embolism (PE), embolisation to the lungs, which is a potentially fatal condition. In the UK, the National Institute for Health and Care Excellence (NICE) has published guidance on assessing and reducing the risk of VTE, including DVT and PE, in hospitalised patients (NICE 2018). These guidelines identify people most at risk and describe interventions to reduce VTE. Risk factors for VTE are outlined in Table 53.1.

Influencing Factors

When considering the how and the when of a VTE assessment, the healthcare profession needs to be mindful of the certain key points:

- All adult patients should be VTE risk-assessed as soon as possible after admission or in pre-assessment clinic (NICE 2018) with the assessment decision reviewed by a senior clinician as per local policy.
- Reassessment should take place within 24 hours of admission and following any clinical changes. This should consider the suitability of the chosen method of VTE prophylaxis and whether it is being used appropriately.
- Patients should also be informed about the correct use of VTE prophylaxis, such as anti-embolism stockings, intermittent pneumatic compression, or pharmacological investigations with a rationale provided for the method used.
- When pharmacological thromboprophylaxis is prescribed, the clinical judgement of a senior clinician is required to balance risk of VTE against risk of bleeding.
- Pharmacological thromboprophylaxis should be started within 14 hours of admission.

Professional Approach

- Patient-informed consent must be obtained prior to conducting the VTE assessment.
- The patient must be made aware of their level of VTE risk and the options available to reduce this risk, including education on hydration and early mobilisation.
- Selection of the most appropriate thromboprophylaxis should consider patient preference.
- All patients at increased risk of VTE should be given written information about the risks and consequences of VTE, as well as the possible side-effects of VTE prophylaxis, such as bleeding.

Equipment

A risk assessment tool should be used to guide the identification of VTE risk (DH 2018) (Table 53.2). This form will help in selecting the most appropriate method of thromboprophylaxis for that individual (Muñoz-Figueroa and Ojo 2015). Generally, the form used will be local to the clinical organisation.

Procedure

- With their consent, assess the patient using a validated VTE risk assessment tool as per local policy.

- First, assess their level of mobility. All surgical patients and medical patients expected to have reduced mobility relative to their normal state will require further assessment of their thrombosis and bleeding risks.
- Assess for thrombosis risk, both patient- and procedure-related.
- Any identified thrombosis risk should prompt the commencement of thromboprophylaxis (NICE 2018).
- Assess for bleeding risk, both patient- and procedure-related.
- Where a factor related to bleeding risk has been identified, the clinician must consider if this is enough to prevent pharmacological intervention.
- Thromboprophylaxis must be prescribed – chemical, mechanical or a combination of both.
- Any contraindications to thromboprophylaxis must be documented in the medical notes.
- Any change in patient VTE risk must be documented and rationale given for alteration to thromboprophylaxis.
- If the patient is being discharged or transferred to another care provider on extended thromboprophylaxis, this must be documented in the notes and the GP or care facility informed.
- The patient and/or carer must then be given verbal and written information on intended duration and side-effects.
- Their understanding and level of skill in administration of the thromboprophylaxis must then be assessed.
- On discharge patients/carers should be offered verbal and written information on VTE prevention and the recognition of symptoms should they occur.

NB: VTE prophylaxis is either mechanical (e.g. anti-embolism stockings) or pharmacological (e.g. anticoagulants such as low-molecular-weight heparin [LMWH]), or both.

Red Flags

- ☛ Despite VTE prophylaxis the nurse must remain vigilant for the signs and symptoms of DVT and PE.
- ☛ Pharmacological VTE prophylaxis carries a small risk of bleeding and the nurse should look out for signs of bleeding or bruising.

References

Department of Health (2018) *Risk Assessment for Venous Thromboembolism (VTE)*. www.nice.org.uk/guidance/ng89/resources/department-of-health-vte-risk-assessment-tool-pdf-4787149213 (accessed on 30 November 2020).

Muñoz-Figueroa, G.P. and Ojo, O. (2015). Venous thromboembolism: use of graduated compression stockings. *British Journal of Nursing*. 24 (13): 680–685.

National Institute of Health and Care Excellence (2018) *Guideline NG 89: Venous Thromboembolism in Over 16s: Reducing the Risk of Hospital-acquired Deep Vein Thrombosis or Pulmonary Embolism*. www.nice.org.uk/guidance/ng89/resources/venous-thromboembolism-in-over-16s-reducing-the-risk-of-hospitalacquired-deep-vein-thrombosis-or-pulmonary-embolism-pdf-1837703092165 (accessed on 30 November 2020).

NHS Digital (2020) *Deaths from Venous Thromboembolism (VTE) Related Events Within 90 Days Post Discharge from Hospital*. https://digital.nhs.uk/data-and-information/publications/statistical/nhs-outcomes-framework/august-2020/domain-5-treating-and-caring-for-people-in-a-safe-environment-and-protecting-them-from-avoidable-harm-nof/5-1-deaths-from-venous-thromboembolism-vte-related-events-within-90-days-post-discharge-from-hospital (accessed on 30 November 2020).

54 Anti-embolic stockings

Table 54.1 Contraindications to anti-embolic stockings (AES).

Patients who should not be offered AES are those who have:

* Peripheral arterial occlusive disease

* Peripheral arterial bypass grafting

* Peripheral neuropathy

* Any local skin conditions such as fragile skin, dermatitis, gangrene, or recent skin graft

* Known allergy to material of manufacture

* Severe leg oedema

* Extreme leg deformity or unusual leg shape preventing correct fit

* Thigh circumference that exceeds manufacturer's specifications.

Figure 54.1 Measuring legs.

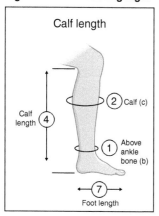
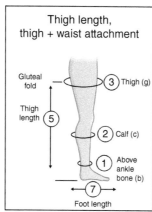

Calf length

Thigh length, thigh + waist attachment

Calf length ④

② Calf (c)

① Above ankle bone (b)

⑦ Foot length

Gluteal fold

Thigh length ⑤

③ Thigh (g)

② Calf (c)

① Above ankle bone (b)

⑦ Foot length

Figure 54.2 Place hand inside stocking to heel.

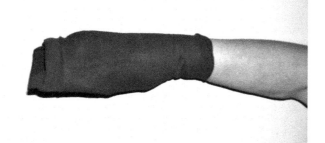

Figure 54.3 Ensure that heel is fitted correctly.

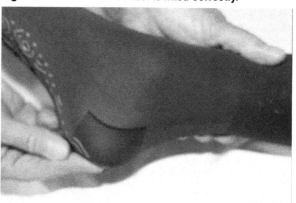

Figure 54.4 Correct placement with two finger measurements.

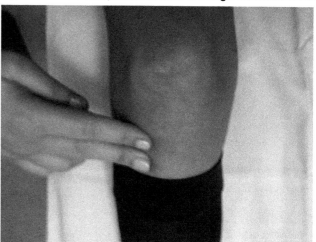

Table 54.2 Anti-embolic stockings (AES) – discharge information (NICE 2018).

Ensure that people who are discharged home with anti-embolism stockings:

* Understand why they need to wear them

* Understand how to wear them correctly

* Understand the need to remove them daily for hygiene purposes

* Have a spare pair to enable them to be washed

* Can remove and replace them, or have someone who can do this for them

* Know to examine their skin for any marking, blistering or discoloration, particularly over the heels and bony prominences

* Have contact details for someone if they have a problem

* Know how long they need to wear them.

Clinical Nursing Skills at a Glance, First Edition. Edited by Sarah Curr and Carol Fordham-Clarke.
© 2022 John Wiley & Sons Ltd. Published 2022 by John Wiley & Sons Ltd.
Companion website: www.wiley.com/go/clinicalnursingskills

Background

Prophylaxis against venous thromboembolism (VTE) is an important part of the nursing role and can be achieved via mechanical or pharmacological methods. Anti-embolic stockings (AES), sometimes called graduated compression stockings, are the most common method of mechanical thromboprophylaxis used (Muñoz-Figueroa and Ojo 2015). They are offered to those patients identified as at increased risk in a VTE risk assessment (Chapter 53).

Anti-embolic stockings work by reducing the cross-sectional area of the limb, thus compressing the deep veins. This assists venous return by increasing venous blood flow velocity, preventing venous dilation and stasis. Anti-embolic stockings deliver a graduated pressure pattern, which is highest in the ankle region (18 mmHg), 14 mmHg in the calf, and lowest in the upper thigh region (8 mmHg), thereby applying a pressure which gradually decreases up the leg (Macintyre et al. 2016). Both knee and thigh length stockings are available.

Influencing Factors

- Measurement of the legs should preferably be taken early in the morning and with the patient lying down, as patient position and time of day may affect the shape and size of the leg.
- A single-patient-use tape measure should be used to measure the legs to prevent cross-infection.
- AES must be prescribed by a doctor or non-medical prescriber following VTE risk assessment.
- The patient should be provided with written information about VTE and the use of AES to prevent this.
- The practitioner must be aware of the contraindications to the application of AES (Table 54.1).
- AES should be worn continuously and only removed for personal hygiene for no longer than 30 minutes or as per local policy.

Professional Approach

- Nurses involved in the fitting and application of AES must have received training and be assessed as competent.
- Prior to applying AES, patients should be assessed for suitability and any contraindications to their use documented.
- Informed consent must be provided to fitting and wearing the stockings, to ensure that the patient understands the rationale for use and that adequate compliance is achieved.
- Ensure patient privacy and dignity are preserved while measuring for and fitting the AES.

Equipment

- Prescription for AES.
- Single-patient-use tape measure.
- Manufacturer sizing chart.
- VTE and AES patient information leaflets, if available.

Procedure – Measuring the Legs

- Perform hand hygiene and put on personal protective equipment, if required.
- With the patient lying down, expose the legs by removing socks, tights, and trousers if applying thigh-length stockings.
- Measure both the patient's legs according to the manufacturer's guidelines (Figure 54.1).
- Where measurements from each leg are different, two different sizes of stocking are needed to ensure the correct fit on each leg.
- Check for any patient allergy or sensitivity to any of the components of the stockings.

Procedure – Applying the Stockings

To fit knee-length stockings:

- Ensure the patient's feet and legs are clean and dry. Dusting the legs and feet with talcum powder can help to slide the stockings on.
- Put the hand inside the stocking as far as the heel pocket (Figure 54.2).
- Grasping the centre of the heel pocket., pull the stocking inside-out to the heel area.
- Place the stocking over the foot, ensuring that the heel is correctly fitted (Figure 54.3).
- Taking the excess stocking at the front of the foot, pull the body of the stocking up around the ankle and onwards over the calf.
- Smooth out any excess material.
- Ensure the top of stocking is about two fingers' width below the crease of the knee (Figure 54.4).

To fit thigh-length stockings:

- As above – then pull the stocking over the calf and subsequently over the knee, ensuring that the non-graduated knee area is in place.
- Pull the remainder of the stocking over the thigh, ensuring that the top band sits in the upper thigh area directly below the buttocks and that the gusset is over the inner thigh.

For both lengths of stocking:

- Smooth out any wrinkles, pulling the toe section forward to smooth the ankle and instep areas.
- Ensure the toes are covered and the open toe is located under the toe area.
- Check that the elastic stocking top is not too tight or too loose, as this indicates incorrect sizing.
- Record the following in the patient's medical notes: leg measurements, and who took them, type and size of stocking, date applied, and intended duration.
- Provide the patient with self-care skills on taking care of their AES, particularly if being discharged home (Table 54.2).

Red Flags

- If oedema or postoperative swelling develops, the legs must be re-measured and stockings refitted.
- Incorrectly fitted AES can result in pressure ulcers on heels and toes, tissue necrosis, and blisters on the skin, which can lead to infection and leg ulcers. Arterial blood flow can be restricted, possibly leading to limb ischaemia.
- Do not allow stockings to roll down the leg, creating a tourniquet effect that exerts greater pressure around the leg, resulting in skin damage and reduced venous velocity.
- Stockings can be slippery underfoot and mobile patients must be encouraged to wear footwear to prevent falls.
- Should the patient complain that the stockings are too tight or causing pain, immediately remove the AES, and check the skin for limb ischaemia and skin integrity.

References

Macintyre, L., Stewart, H., and Rae, M. (2016). How can the pressure in anti-embolism stockings be maintained during use? Laboratory evaluation of simulated 'wear' and different reconditioning protocols. *International Journal of Nursing Studies* 65: 19–24.

Muñoz-Figueroa, G.P. and Ojo, O. (2015). Venous thromboembolism: use of graduated compression stockings. *British Journal of Nursing* 24 (13): 680–685.

National Institute for Health and Care Excellence (2018) *Guideline NG 89: Venous Thromboembolism in Over 16s: Reducing the Risk of Hospital-acquired Deep Vein Thrombosis or Pulmonary Embolism.* www.nice.org.uk/guidance/ng89/resources/venous-thromboembolism-in-over-16s-reducing-the-risk-of-hospitalacquired-deep-vein-thrombosis-or-pulmonary-embolism-pdf-1837703092165 (accessed on 30 November 2020).

55 Musculoskeletal minor injuries: assessment and treatment

Figure 55.1   Triangular bandage sling.

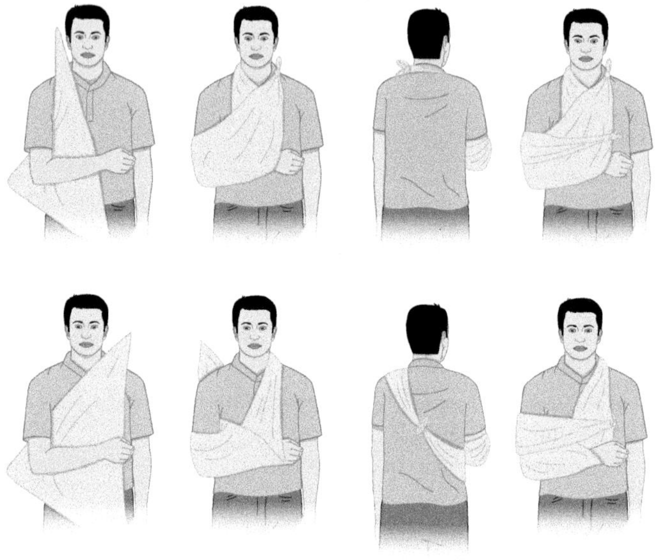

Figure 55.2   Soft tissue injury support.

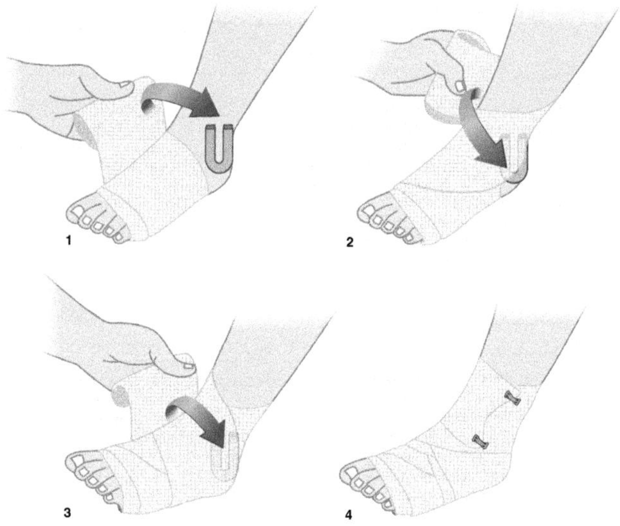

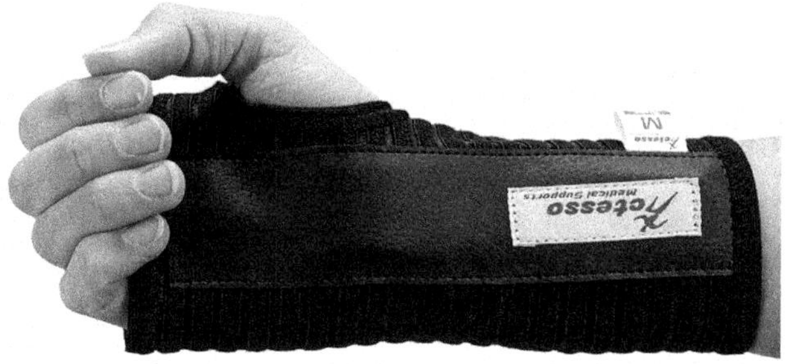

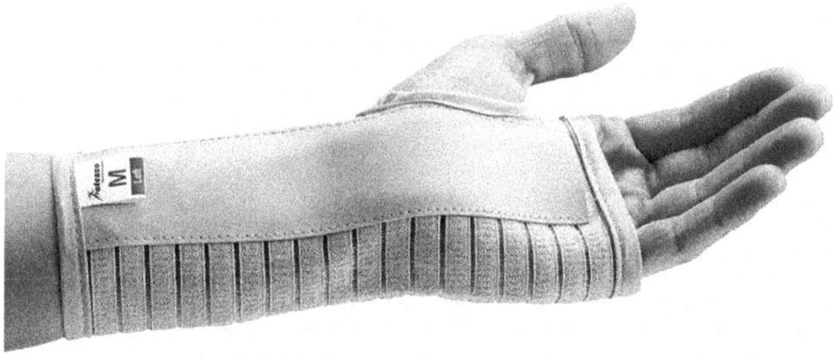

Table 55.1 The Enhanced Calgary-Cambridge Model. Source: Adapted from Kurtz *et al*. (2003).

Initiate the interview	• Establish rapport • Establish the reason for consultation/the injury
Gather information	Explore the issues from the following perspectives: • biomedical • patient • patient information
Physical examination	
Explanation and planning	• Provide appropriate information • Ensure recall and understanding • Ensure a shared understanding • Form shared decision making
Close the session	• Close at appropriate point • Ensure forward planning/next steps

Source: Adapted from Kurtz *et al*. (2003).

Clinical Nursing Skills at a Glance, First Edition. Edited by Sarah Curr and Carol Fordham-Clarke.
© 2022 John Wiley & Sons Ltd. Published 2022 by John Wiley & Sons Ltd.
Companion website: www.wiley.com/go/clinicalnursingskills

Background

Approximately 30–50% of minor musculoskeletal (MSK) injuries seen in primary care are soft tissue injuries, such as sprains and strains (NICE 2016). These also present to the emergency department and urgent care centres and, as such, healthcare professionals working in these areas may well be trained on taking a comprehensive clinical history, determining a diagnosis, and ensuring that appropriate treatment is provided. The focus of this chapter will be on the assessment of MSK minor injuries, the structure of a clinical consultation, and the treatment of soft tissue injuries.

Influencing Factors

- Always ensure that there is enough time to complete the task – both for staff and for the patient.
- Not all MSK injuries will be acute. Chronic MSK injuries could result from work postures as well as repetition of movement, commonly resulting in repetitive strain injury (RSI).

Professional Approach

- Ensure informed consent is obtained.
- Maintain privacy and dignity.
- Effective communication and teamwork are vital during these procedures.
- Provide reassurance and, where possible, involve the patient.
- All individuals should work within their sphere of competence for the safety of all involved.

Equipment

- For all consultations, local policy should be followed, i.e. the Enhanced Calgary-Cambridge Model (Kurtz et al. 2003) (Table 55.1).
- Depending on treatment equipment may include:
  - Analgesics.
  - Anti-inflammatories.
  - Limb or joint support equipment.

Procedure – Clinical Consultation

It is recognised that the clinical assessment is a key component of the consultation (Silverston 2014). The consultation will involve:

- Ascertaining the presenting complaint.
- Gathering information such as mechanism of injury, past medical history, previous injuries, and medication.
- Undertaking a physical examination.
- Considering pain, nociceptive or neuropathic.
- Considering loss of function, neurological or secondary to pain.
- Using specific tools to determine or rule out a fracture.
- Diagnosing the injury and planning the treatment.

NB: The Enhanced Calgary-Cambridge Model (Kurtz et al. 2003) is commonly used in practice as it offers a systematic approach to taking a history for minor injuries (Gloster and Ganley 2012) and, as such, core information on how to use this has been provided in Table 55.1.

Procedure – Clinical Examination

Clinical management of a MSK injury is dependent on the nature and presentation of the injury. A look, listen, move, and feel approach is generally recommended, looking for:

- Swelling, bruising.
- Loss of function.
- Range of movement.
- Heat.
- Bony tenderness – if felt an X-ray may well be indicated.

NB: If a ligament tear is expected a magnetic resonance imaging (MRI) may be required (Gloster and Ganley 2012).

Procedure – First Aid Treatment

For soft tissue injuries, simple analgesia and/or anti-inflammatories need to be offered to the patient, as well as advice regarding PRICE (NICE 2016). PRICE is as follows:

Protection of the injured area.
Resting the injured area.
Ice or other cold compress to the injured area.
Compression to the injured area, not tight.
Elevation of the injured area.

NB: After three days this should be changed to MICE with "M" replacing the "PR" and the patient mobilising.

Procedure – Limb and/or Joint Support

- A sling may be used for certain shoulder and arm injuries/fractures and this must be applied correctly, depending on the injury and management plan for maximum support (Figure 55.1).
- Compression is often required for a soft tissue injury due to the comfort and support it provides (Hansrani et al. 2015) and this may involve an elastic tubular, a compression bandage, or other support (Figure 55.2).

Procedure – Advice for Patients

It is recommended that the term "do no HARM" is used with HARM being followed in the first 48 hours post-injury:

- Heat – avoid heat as swelling may increase due to heat induced vasodilation.
- Alcohol – affects coordination, potentially leading to further injury.
- Running – this increases blood flow to the area and can increase oedema and the potential for haemorrhage or further injury to the area.
- Massage – this also increases circulation to the area and will exacerbate oedema and swelling.

Red Flags

☛ If a suspicious injury is suspected, the process for safeguarding children, vulnerable adults, or elderly must be followed.

☛ Fractures must be ruled out prior to soft tissue injury treatment and discharge advice. These will require specialist management and care.

☛ Immediate care must be provided if there are signs of decreased circulation to the affected area.

References

Gloster, A. and Ganley, L. (2012). Care of patients with minor injuries. *Nursing Standard* 26 (21): 50–57.

Hansrani, V., Khanbhai, M., Bahandari, S. et al. (2015). The role of compression in the management of soft tissue ankle injuries: a systematic review. *European Journal of Orthopaedic Surgery & Traumatology* 25 (6): 987–995.

Kurtz, S.M., Silverman, J.D., Benson, J., and Draper, J. (2003). Marrying content and process in clinical method teaching: enhancing the Calgary-Cambridge guides. *Academic Medicine* 78 (8): 802–809.

National Institute for Health and Care Excellence (2016). *Clinical Knowledge Summary. Sprains and Strains.* https://cks.nice.org.uk/sprains-and-strains (accessed 6 December 2020).

Silverston, P. (2014). The safe clinical assessment: a patient safety focused approach to clinical assessment. *Nurse Education Today* 34 (2): 214–217.

56 Falls – prevention, assessment and management

Table 56.1 Backward chaining.

1	**Position a chair at the head end of the fallen person**	
2	Verbally support the person to bend their knees up and to bring one arm across their chest	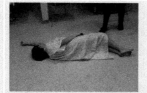
3	Ask the person to roll onto their side	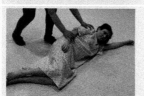
4	Once on the side, ask the person to bring their arm over their body until the hand is flat on the floor	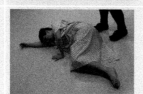
5	Support the person to push up on their hand and at the same time push up on their forearm that is resting on the floor until they are half sitting	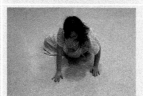
6	Support the person until they end up on all fours and are facing the chair	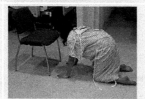
7	Ask the person to position their lower arms on the chair and ask them to lean onto the seat of the chair	
8	Ask the person to raise the stronger leg and place the foot flat on the floor	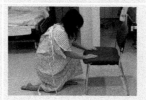

9	The handler inserts another chair under the raised buttock of the person	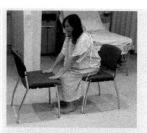
10	The person sits back onto the second chair/wheelchair (with brakes on)	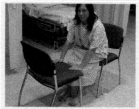

Table 56.2 Rolling a person on the floor to position handling equipment.

1. Ask or assist the person to position the furthest arm across the chest.
2. At the same time, ask or assist the person to bend one or both knees, ensuring that feet are flat on the floor.
3. Bring the nearest arm away from the body and leave flat on the floor, to prevent the person rolling onto their arm or hand.
4. Ask the person to turn their head and face in the direction of the turn.
5. One handler kneels down on both knees and starts off with their heels off the buttocks, high kneeling.
6. At the same time the handler holds the person's hip and shoulder.
7. The handler brings the hips and shoulders over as they sit back onto their heels, low kneeling.
8. Once the equipment (i.e. sling) has been fitted, roll the person onto their back and repeat on the other side.

Table 56.3 Managing a confined space fall.

1. After completing an assessment of the person and the environment, the handler should encourage the person to lie flat.
2. The handler takes a transfer sheet and concertinas this up.
3. Two handlers are required from now on.
4. Kneel down beside the person, one at either side.
5. This transfer sheet is inserted under the head end of the person.
6. The two handlers each hold onto the bottom corner strap of the transfer sheet.
7. Pulling all of the time, shimmy this underneath the person down to the ankles and check when the transfer sheet sticks. If the transfer sheet sticks, unstick it.
8. Keep pulling the transfer sheet by the handles until the transfer sheet is all the way under the person.
9. Handlers stand up, have a walk posture and pull the bottom two straps.
10. On a given signal, the handlers should transfer their weight onto the back leg.
11. Instruction is "Ready – steady – pull." Remember that this instruction may have to be continued until the person is in a place of safety.
12. As in all team handling, one handler should be responsible for coordinating the move.

Clinical Nursing Skills at a Glance, First Edition. Edited by Sarah Curr and Carol Fordham-Clarke.
© 2022 John Wiley & Sons Ltd. Published 2022 by John Wiley & Sons Ltd.
Companion website: www.wiley.com/go/clinicalnursingskills

Background

- Maintaining good balance and mobility are central to independence, social connectivity, and well-being in older age (Patel et al. 2014). Age-related changes in sensory and motor systems have an impact on gait and balance, and as such older people are at an increased risk of falls, injury, and negative psychological impacts (Patel et al. 2014).
- Maintaining mobility through building muscle conditioning, strength, and balance training are core to ageing well and reducing risk of falls (Cameron et al. 2018). Nurses across all care settings have the potential to influence older people and their families to ensure prevention of falls and effective assessment and treatment following a fall.

Influencing Factors

A fall will usually occur as a result of:

- Advanced age.
- Limited mobility.
- Medication and polypharmacy.
- Environmental reasons, i.e. home hazards.
- Impaired gait and mobility.

Professional Approach

- Ensure informed consent is obtained.
- Maintain privacy and dignity.
- Effective communication and teamwork are vital during these procedures.
- Provide reassurance and, where possible, involve the patient.
- All individuals should work within their sphere of competence for the safety of all involved.
- Complete the incident form as per institution guidelines and policies.
- Inform the family.

Equipment

Depending on the procedure you will require:

- The appropriate number of competent personnel.
- Sliding sheet.
- Chair.
- Wheelchair.

Procedure – Falls Prevention

- Pro-active case finding.
- Medication review.
- Multifaceted risk assessment.
- Vision assessment and referral.
- Home hazards.
- Strength and balance training.
  (NICE 2013).

Procedure – Post-Fall Procedure

Immediate response:

- DR – ABCDE.
- A – If the patient won't stay on the floor – Assist from the floor, can patient get up themselves?
- M – Monitor neuro-observations.
- A – Act if any concerns.
- C – Contact family.
- Check for injuries – if no apparent injury assist patient to bed or chair (Table 56.1).

  NB: If there are signs of head injury, fracture/deformity, seek medical assistance.

Procedure – Post-Fall Interventions

- Perform vital and neurological observations.
- Multidisciplinary team review to consider cause of fall and action required.
- Medication review.
- Investigate medical causes, including tests of urine, lying and standing blood pressure, temperature, electrocardiogram (ECG).
- Refer to physiotherapy for assessment/review of the service user's balance and mobility, and provide appropriate advice and/or mobility aids; evidence-based exercise programmes for fall prevention may be indicated.
- Refer to occupational therapy for assessment of the safest ways for individuals to carry out activities of daily living, if indicated.
- Communicate the advice from physiotherapy and occupational therapy to all staff, and ensure mobility aids remain within reach.
- Assess the service user's continence. Consider referral to continence nurse specialist or urological services if increased urgency resulted in the fall.
- Undertake an osteoporotic risk factors review and, if necessary, treat/request GP intervention (as per NICE 2016).
- Consider use of bed rails using identified tool; review is a complex issue especially in mental health units. Always follow local policy.

Procedure – Backward Chaining

- Assess whether the person:
  - can be verbally instructed.
  - has the physical ability to roll to their side and onto all fours.
- Follow step-by-step instructions in Table 56.1.

Procedure – Rolling a Person on the Floor to Position Handling Equipment

- Assess whether the person can assist with the transfer or requires full assistance.
- Follow the steps outlined in Table 56.2.

Procedure – Managing a Confined Space Fall

- Assess whether the person can assist with the transfer.
- Follow the technique outline in Table 56.3 to support a person to roll over, get onto all fours, and return to a chair.

Red Flags

- ☛ Serious injuries – ensure a thorough assessment before supporting the person to mobilise.
- ☛ Monitor for possible clinical deterioration.

References

Cameron, I.D., Dyer, S.M., Panagoda, C.E., Murray, G.R., Hill, K.D., Cumming, R.G. & Kerse, N. (2018) *Interventions for Preventing Falls in Older People in Care Facilities and Hospitals.* Cochrane Database of Systematic Reviews. https://www.cochrane.org/CD005465/MUSKINJ_interventions-preventing-falls-older-people-care-facilities-and-hospitals (accessed 22 May 2021).

National Institute of Health and Care Excellence (2013) *Falls in Older People: Assessing Risk and Prevention. Clinical Guideline [CG161].* www.nice.org.uk/guidance/cg161 (accessed 22 May 2021).

National Institute of Health and Care Excellence (2016) *Osteoporosis – Prevention of Fragility Fractures.* https://cks.nice.org.uk/topics/osteoporosis-prevention-of-fragility-fractures (accessed 22 May 2021).

Patel, K.V., Phelan, E.A., Leveille, S.G. et al. (2014). High prevalence of falls, fear of falling, and impaired balance in older adults with pain in the United States: findings from the 2011 National Health and aging trends study. *Journal of the American Geriatrics Society* 62 (10): 1844–1852.

57 Stabilisation: neck collar

Table 57.1 Checks for sensory and motor function as well as positional awareness in all limbs.

Sensory and Motor Assessment		
Nerve	**Sensory**	**Motor**
C2	At least 1 cm lateral to occipital protuberance at base of skull; can also be located at least 3 cm behind ear	Respiration
C3	In supraclavicular fossa at midclavicular line	
C4	Over acromioclavicular joint	
C5	On lateral (radial) side of antecubital fossa just proximal to elbow	Elbow flexion (biceps)
C6	On dorsal surface of proximal phalanx of thumb	Wrist extension (extensor carpi radialis)
C7	On dorsal surface of proximal phalanx of middle finger	Elbow extension (triceps)
C8	On dorsal surface of proximal phalanx of little finger	Long finger flexion (flexor digitorum profundus)
T1	On medial (ulnar) side of the antecubital fossa, just proximal to medial epicondyle of humerus	Small finger abduction (abductor digiti minimi)
T2	At apex of axilla	Posture, respiration support
T3	At midclavicular line and third intercostal space; found by palpating anteriorchest to locate third rib and corresponding third intercostal space below it	
T4	At midclavicular line and fourth intercostal space; located at level of nipples	
T5	At midclavicular line and fifth intercostal space; located midway between level of nipples and level of xiphisternum	
T6	At midclavicular line, located at level of xiphisternum	
T7	At midclavicular line, one-quarter the distance between level of xiphisternum and level of umbilicus	
T8	At midclavicular line, half the distance between level of xiphisternum and level of umbilicus	
T9	At midclavicular line, three-quarters the distance between level of xiphisternum and level of umbilicus	
T10	At midclavicular line, located at level of umbilicus	
T11	At midclavicular line, midway between level of umbilicus and inguinal ligament	
T12	At midclavicular line, over midpoint of inguinal ligament	
L1	Midway between key sensory points for T12 and L2	
L2	On anteromedial thigh, at midpoint drawn on an imaginary line connecting midpoint of inguinal ligament and medial femoral condyle	Hip flexion (iliopsoas)
L3	At medial femoral condyle above knee	Knee extension (quadriceps)
L4	Over medial malleolus	Ankle dorsiflexion (tibialis anterior)
L5	On dorsum of foot at third metatarsophalangeal joint	Great toe extension (extensor hallucis longus)
S1	On lateral aspect of calcaneus	Ankle plantarflexion (gastrocnemius, soleus)
S2	At midpoint of popliteal fossa	
S3	Over ischial tuberosity or intergluteal fold (depending on patient, skin can move up, down or laterally over ischii)	
S4,S5	In perianal area, < 1 cm lateral to mucocutaneous junction.	

Figure 57.1 Measure the patient's neck against anatomical landmarks.

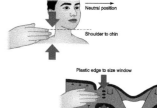

Figure 57.2 Apply the collar while maintaining neutral head position.

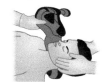

Figure 57.3 Bring the front of the collar into position and fasten the Velcro strap.

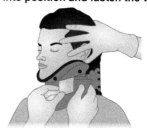

Figure 57.4 Assessing level of lesion.

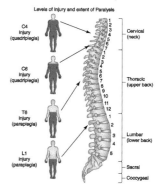

Figure 57.5 Stabilise head with forearms either side.

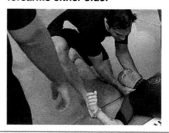

Clinical Nursing Skills at a Glance, First Edition. Edited by Sarah Curr and Carol Fordham-Clarke.
© 2022 John Wiley & Sons Ltd. Published 2022 by John Wiley & Sons Ltd.
Companion website: www.wiley.com/go/clinicalnursingskills

Background

Most spinal cord injuries (SCIs) are associated with injuries to the vertebral column, including fractures, dislocations, and subluxations. High cervical cord transections (above C4) results in loss of respiratory control and death if not promptly recognised and treated appropriately (Alizadeh et al. 2019).

Approximately 53% of SCI cases involve adolescents or young adults aged 16–30 years; most injuries are caused by motor vehicle crashes, falls, violence (such as gunshot wounds), and sports (WHO 2013). As such patients with a suspected spinal injury will require a full neurological assessment (Chapters 17 and 18) and specific care to ensure spine immobilisation (Alizadeh et al. 2019).

In a diagnosed SCI, the primary goal is to preserve or improve neurological function (Alizadeh et al. 2019). Treatment is thus focused on prevention of secondary injury, spinal realignment, and stabilisation, as well as prevention of complications.

Influencing Factors

Spinal cord injuries commonly result from a sudden, traumatic impact on the spine that fractures or dislocates vertebrae. The initial mechanical forces delivered to the spinal cord at the time of injury is called the primary injury (Alizadeh et al. 2019).

Professional Approach

- Ensure informed consent is obtained.
- Maintain privacy and dignity.
- Effectively communicate within the team.
- Provide reassurance and, where possible, involve the patient in the decision-making.
- Ensure all individuals are working within their sphere of competence.

Equipment

Depending on the procedure you will require:

- Appropriate number of competent personnel.
- Neck collar.

Procedure – Application of a One-Piece Collar

Whilst neck collar use is being debated (Sundstrøm et al. 2014; Hodgett and Ward 2020) they are currently still in use and local policy should be followed. Do also ensure that a suitable trained and experienced healthcare professional performs the following:

- Explain what is happening, why, and next steps.
- Check sensory and motor function as well as positional awareness in all limbs (Table 57.1).
- Measure the patient's neck against anatomical landmarks (Figure 57.1).
- Adjust the collar to the appropriate size.
- Ensure the collar is fitted to bare skin for a secure position. Clothing may need to be cut away and jewellery removed.
- With a trained professional holding the patient's head secure (Chapter 58), an assistant feeds the back piece of the collar into position, pressing the collar into the mattress surface to prevent friction with the patient's skin (Figure 57.2).
- Another assistant then manoeuvres the collar into the correct position ensuring that as much of the head is encompassed as possible ensuring that the ears are not obscured.
- Then bring the front of the collar into position and fasten the Velcro strap (Figure 57.3).
- Check sensory and motor function as well as positional awareness in all limbs again (Table 57.1).
- The healthcare professional holding the head and shoulders can now release.

Procedure – Application of a Two-Piece Collar

A two-piece collar provides continued spinal protection in patients with actual or suspected cervical spinal or SCI. The two-piece collar should replace the pre-hospital collar to reduce the risk of pressure ulcers and venous obstruction (Sarhan et al. 2013). Steps that a trained and experienced healthcare professional takes are as follows:

- Follow initial steps of application of a one-piece collar.
- Once the collar is in position, the front piece of the collar is brought up and underneath the chin in a straight line.
- Then fasten the Velcro before checking sensory and motor functions as well as positional awareness in all limbs again (Table 57.1).

NB: Curling and flexing of the collar piece before fitting ensures a more comfortable fit.

Procedure – Adapted Advanced Trauma Life Support Head Hold for Actual or Potential Cervical Spinal Injury

1 Ensure that a trained and competent individual has assessed the level of the lesion (cervical, thoracic, lumbar, or sacrum; Figure 57.4).
2 Explain to the patient what is happening and why.
3 Designate a suitably qualified healthcare professional as team leader. The team leader will stand at the top of the trolley/bed, placing hands either side of patient's head.
4 The team leader then spreads fingers wide and slides both hands downwards so the thumb rests either below the jaw or above the clavicle and the fingers are spread behind the neck at C7.
5 If sandbags/headblocks are present, an assistant removes them, one at a time, and the team leader brings each hand into position individually.
6 Forearms are then brought together either side at the back of the head (Figure 57.5).
7 Ensure that the bed is at an adequate height to prevent excessive forward trunk flexion of the team leader.
8 Roll the patient on the team leader's command. To accommodate this roll, the team leader may be required to adopt a side flexed position.
9 To ensure a comfortable head hold during the log roll, the team leader releases their top hand and moves the hand slowly to the top of the patient's head with fingers spread wide. They then adjust their base of support to a more comfortable/sustainable position while keeping the head in the aligned position.

NB: The team leader can be provided a chair during prolonged holding, with the elbows then resting on a pillow. In patients with broad shoulders, a pillow or pad can also be used to support the team leader's underlying arm, but it must be of the correct depth to maintain spinal alignment.

Red Flags

☞ An improperly placed neck collar can cause more damage to the cervical spine.

References

Alizadeh, A., Dyck, S.M., and Karimi-Abdolrezaee, S. (2019). Traumatic spinal cord injury: an overview of pathophysiology, models and acute injury mechanisms. *Frontiers in Neurology* 10 (282): 1–25.

Hodgett, R. and Ward, R. (2020). Are cervical collars effective and safe in prehospital spinal cord injury management? *Journal of Paramedic Medicine* 12 (2): 67–78.

Sarhan, F., Saif, D., and Saif, A. (2013). An overview of traumatic spinal cord injury: part 2. Acute management. *British Journal of Neuroscience Nursing* 9 (3): 138–144.

Sundstrøm, T., Asbjørnsen, H., Habiba, S. et al. (2014). Prehospital use of cervical collars in trauma patients: a critical review. *Journal of Neurotrauma* 31 (6): 531–540.

World Health Organization. *Spinal Cord Injury*. Factsheet no. 384. (2013). https://www.who.int/news-room/fact-sheets/detail/spinal-cord-injury (accessed 6 December 2020).

58 Care of the patient with spinal cord injuries – log roll

Figure 58.1 (a) Fifth assistant position (front, centre) for tetraplegic spinal log roll. (b) Patient's arms positioned across the chest but above the diaphragm.

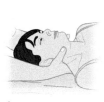

1.

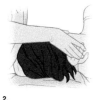

2.

3.

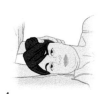

4.

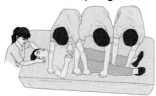

Figure 58.3 Third assistant position, tetraplegic spinal log roll; second assistant position, paraplegic spinal log roll.

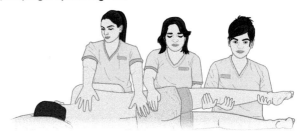

Figure 58.2 Second assistant position, tetraplegic spinal log roll; first assistant position, paraplegic spinal log roll.

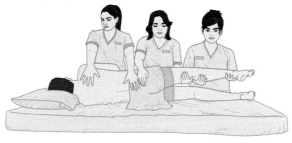

Figure 58.4 Fourth assistant position, tetraplegic spinal log roll; third assistant position, paraplegic spinal log roll.

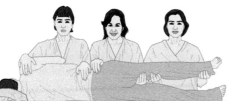

Figure 58.5 Pillow support in a side position.

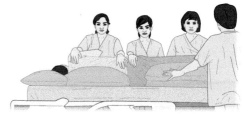

Figure 58.6 Floating heels.

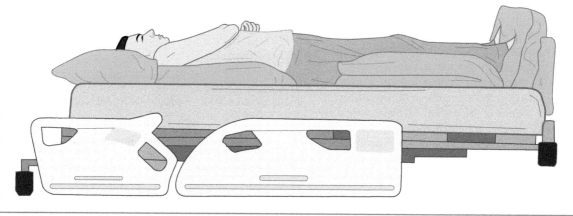

Clinical Nursing Skills at a Glance, First Edition. Edited by Sarah Curr and Carol Fordham-Clarke.
© 2022 John Wiley & Sons Ltd. Published 2022 by John Wiley & Sons Ltd.
Companion website: www.wiley.com/go/clinicalnursingskills

Background

With suspected or confirmed spinal injuries it is essential to protect the spine (Maschmann et al. 2019). As highlighted in Chapter 57 a neck collar will often be applied. In instances where the patient needs to be moved, such as for relieving pressure on the skin, hygiene, and bowel care, a log roll will need to be undertaken until a spinal injury is ruled out.

Influencing Factors

A log roll will need to be performed by trained personnel with an experienced member of staff as team leader. Prior to undertaking the log roll, a patient's ability to tolerate the procedure needs to be considered.

Professional Approach

Prior to performing a log roll the following are essential:

- Explain the process to the patient and make sure it is understood, in order to ensure informed consent.
- Consider the patient's privacy and dignity.
- Speak to and reassure the patient about the procedure – this must be continued throughout.

Equipment

- Necessary personnel (depending on the manoeuvre this can be either four to five people).
- A designated team leader.

Procedure – Acute Tetraplegic Spinal Log Roll

Log rolling on a trolley in the emergency department or within a ward setting on a normal hospital bed or tilt-and-turn bed is essential to enable examination of the back and necessary for relieving pressure on the skin, hygiene, bowel care, and postural chest drainage. The following technique is suggested by the Multidisciplinary Association of Spinal Cord Injury Professionals (MASCIP 2015) and is applicable in all clinical settings:

1 The first assistant/team leader undertakes acute initial head hold in accordance with adapted Advanced Trauma Life Support (ATLS) procedure (Chapter 57).
2 The fifth assistant passively positions the patient's arms across the chest but above the diaphragm (Figure 58.1). This is important as the arms are paralysed and may fall, causing injury to the shoulder joint.
3 The second assistant reaches over the patient and places their first hand on the shoulder and their second hand on top of the hip (Figure 58.2). The fifth assistant also supports the patient's arm during this action.
4 The third assistant positions the first hand at hip level alongside the second assistant, and the second hand underneath the furthest thigh (Figure 58.3).
5 The fourth assistant positions the first hand under the knee of the furthest leg, and the second hand under the ankle of the same leg (Figure 58.4).
6 Ensure that all parties are in contact with the patient's natural skeletal landmarks and not just adipose tissue.

Procedure – Acute Paraplegic Spinal Log Roll

This log rolling procedure is also suggested by MASCIP (2015) and is undertaken in acute paraplegic patients in whom the possibility of accompanying cervical spinal injury has been excluded. This log roll only requires four healthcare professionals as patients can support and control their own head movements. It is performed as follows:

1 Following a risk assessment a single pillow can be placed under the head for patients demonstrating spondylitis.
2 The first assistant reaches over the patient and places their first hand on the shoulder and their second hand on the top of the hip (Figure 58.2).
3 The second assistant positions the first hand at hip level alongside the first assistant, and the second hand underneath the furthest thigh (Figure 58.3).
4 The third assistant position places the first hand under the knee of the furthest leg, and the second hand under the ankle of the same leg (Figure 58.4).
5 The log roll is performed under the team leader's instruction.
6 Following the log roll, the patient's upper leg must be kept in alignment with the lower leg throughout the turn to prevent any flexion movement being relayed to the thoraco-lumbar spine. To maintain lateral alignment, the outer malleolus should be maintained at a height level with the upper trochanter (Figure 58.4).
7 With the patient supported in a log roll, one pillow is then placed to support the patient's back.
8 Two pillows can be positioned to support the upper leg in a side-lying position (Figure 58.5).

   NB: Ensure that legs are positioned to prevent hyperextension of the knees – a bed end is placed in situ and additional pillows are placed at the end of the bed to support the patient's feet in neutral to prevent foot drop. The heels are left "floating" free from pressure to prevent skin breakdown (Figure 58.6).

Red Flags

- Signs of breathlessness and chest pain, worse on inspiration, could indicate a pulmonary embolism and must be escalated and managed immediately.
- Severe headache, hypertension, bradycardia, nasal congestion, blurred vision, anxiety/distress, nausea, flushing of the head/neck, and diaphoresis above the lesion could suggest autonomic dysreflexia and the underlying cause must be identified and removed.
- Do not transport people with acute spinal cord injury (National Institute of Health and Care Excellence 2016).

References

Maschmann, C., Jeppesen, E., Rubin, M.A., and Barfod, C. (2019). New clinical guidelines on the spinal stabilisation of adult trauma patients – consensus and evidence based. *Scandinaven Journal of Trauma, Resuscitation and Emergency Medicine* 27 (77): 1–10.

Multidisciplinary Association of Spinal Cord Injury Professionals (2015) Moving and Handling of Patients with Actual or Suspected Spinal Cord Injuries (SCI). https://www.mascip.co.uk/wp-content/uploads/2015/02/MASCIP-SIA-Guidelines-for-MH-Trainers.pdf (accessed 23rd June 2021).

National Institute of Health and Care Excellence (2016). *NG41 Spinal Injury: Assessment and Initial Management*. London: National Institute of Health and Care Excellence.

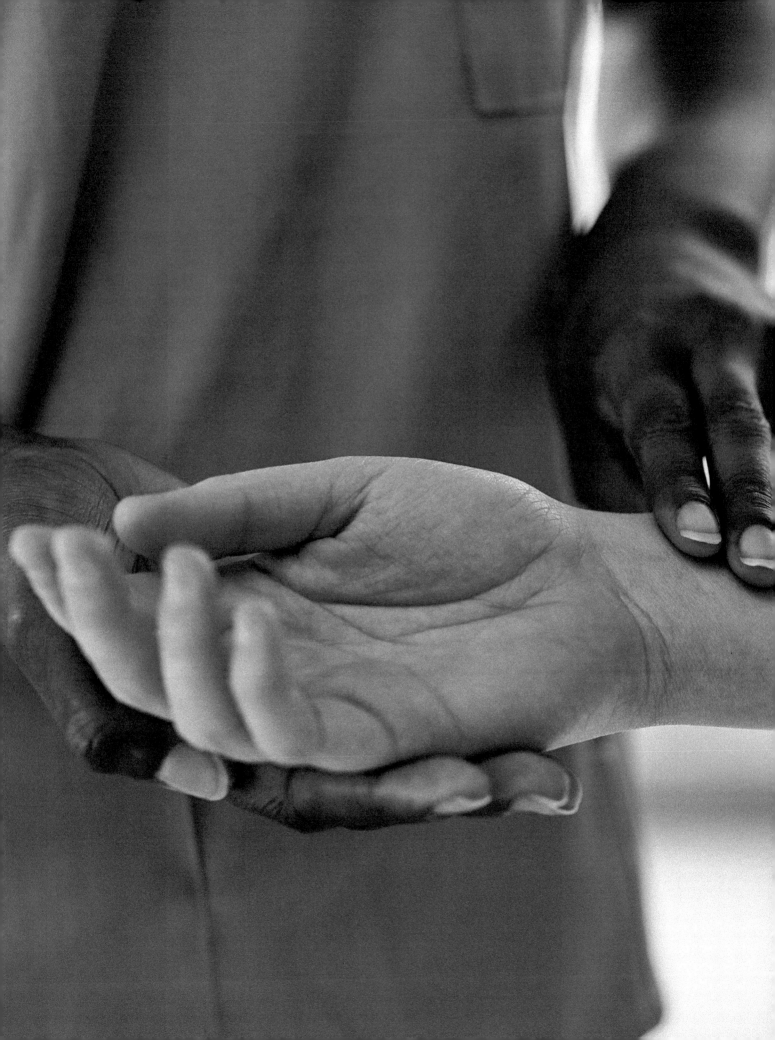

Integumentary skills

Part 10

Chapters

59 Personal hygiene

Figure 59.1   Roll soiled sheet to sacrum.

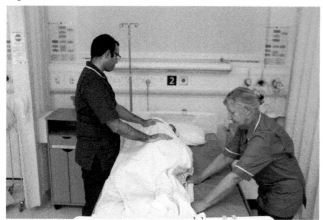

Figure 59.2   Place rolled clean sheet on bed.

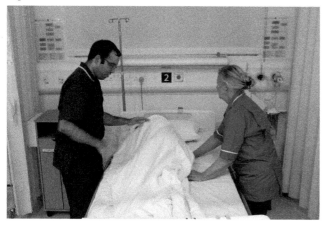

Figure 59.3   Roll patient to other side and remove soiled sheet.

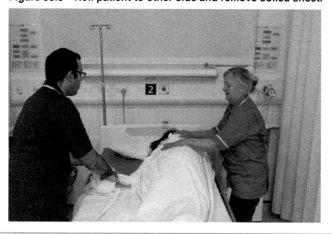

Figure 59.4   Roll out clean sheet and make bed.

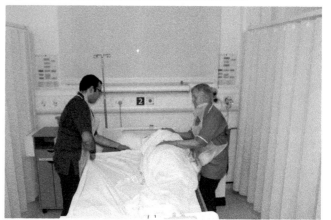

Figure 59.5   Make patient comfortable.

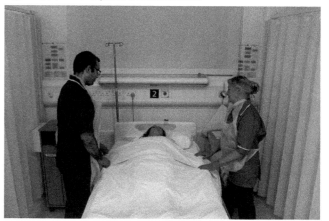

Clinical Nursing Skills at a Glance, First Edition. Edited by Sarah Curr and Carol Fordham-Clarke.
© 2022 John Wiley & Sons Ltd. Published 2022 by John Wiley & Sons Ltd.
Companion website: www.wiley.com/go/clinicalnursingskills

Background

Personal hygiene can be defined as "the physical act of cleansing the body to ensure that the hair, nails, ears, eyes, nose and skin are maintained in optimum condition" (DH 2010, P.183) and support for this is often required in the healthcare setting. As this care will involve support with intimate activities that are usually undertaken independently, sensitivity, respect, and dignity must be maintained.

Influencing Factors

There are many factors that can impact on a person's ability to self-care. These can largely be covered under:

- Individual preference.
- Normal routine.
- Religious traditions.
- Cultural factors.
- Physiological state.
- Psychological state.
- Age.

Professional Approach

- Consider all the above influencing factors and discuss the personal hygiene activities that the patient needs support with before providing personal care.
- Ensure that this conversation occurs on every occasion where personal care is required, as an individual's ability to self-care will vary while receiving care and support with their recovery.

Equipment

Depending on what support is required, equipment could include:

- Bowl – single-use where possible.
- Patient cleansing wipes[1].
- Skin cleansing agent – face and body.
- Moisturisers – face and body.
- Clean towels.
- Clean garments.
- Single-use disposable apron/s and non-sterile gloves.

Procedure – Bed Bath

- Always ascertain if the person can bath or shower with assistance first, as this provides a more thorough cleansing experience.
- Ascertain if the patient requires analgesia or other medication prior to commencing the wash.
- Prepare all the equipment and check the water temperature with the patient before beginning.
- Close the door/curtain and place a do not disturb sign.
- Decontaminate hands and put on apron.
- Ask the patient what they can do themselves and if they are not sure, actively encourage them to perform self-care where able.
- Start with the face, placing a towel under the neck and across the shoulders. Ask the patient to close their eyes and wipe the left eyelid from the inner to the outer corner, pat dry. Repeat with the right eyelid.
- Wash the remainder of the face, ensuring that you also wash and dry behind the ears and neck.

1 These could either be dry or wet wipes.

- Next wash the body from the arm farthest from you, including the axilla.
- Then wash and dry the torso before moving to the arm nearest to you and axilla.

NB: Ensure that you pat dry after each section is cleansed and ascertain if moisturiser or other topical creams or ointments are required and apply. Cover areas not being washed with a towel or sheet.

- Now wash each leg, starting with the leg furthest from you.
- Check the toenails for any signs of abnormality and the skin for dryness, signs of pressure ulcer development, or any other abnormalities.
- Change the water, check the temperature with the patient – if they are to wash their own genitalia, provide them with this opportunity now.
- If the patient is unable to wash this area themselves, decontaminate hands, apply non-sterile gloves, and wash the genitalia from the front to back in females and underneath the foreskin in uncircumcised males.
- Again, change water and check temperature with the patient, decontaminate hands, and reapply non-sterile gloves before assisting the patient onto their side. Cleanse and dry the back before cleansing and drying the sacrum.
- When the patient is on their side, the bottom sheet should be changed by rolling the soiled sheet to the sacrum once cleansing is complete (Figure 59.1) and placing the half-rolled clean sheet on the bed (Figure 59.2). Then roll the patient onto the other side to remove the soiled sheet (Figure 59.3) and unroll the remainder of the clean sheet (Figure 59.4), ensuring that the patient is comfortable (Figure 59.5).
- Dispose of equipment and support the patient in getting dressed, then continue with oral hygiene, hair cleansing, and shaving as required.
- Prior to leaving the patient, ensure that they are seated (or lying) comfortably with the call bell, or other method of contact, within arm's reach.
- Document care provided and other interventions provided.

Red Flags

- A sudden change to the patient's mobility should be fully investigated.
- Any change to skin integrity could indicate pressure ulcer development. Assessment and management should be followed.
- Excessive washing can harm the skin.
- Poor personal hygiene can increase the risk of infection and spread of contagious diseases (Lee et al. 2020).

References
Department of Health (2010). *Essence of Care: Benchmarks for Personal Hygiene*. Norwich: The Stationary Office.

Lee, M.H., Lee, G.A., Lee, S.H., and Park, Y.-H. (2020). A systematic review on the causes of the transmission and control measures of outbreaks in long-term care facilities: back to basics of infection control. *PLoS One* 15 (3): 1–34.

60 Personal hygiene – mouth and hair care

Table 60.1 Oral characteristics – healthy and unhealthy.

Section of the mouth	Healthy characteristics	Unhealthy characteristics
Lips	Smooth and moist	Dry, could also be cracked and bleeding Presence of lesions, ulcers or pustules Abnormal colour
Teeth	Clean, free from plaque Smooth, free from grooves	Discoloured, i.e. yellow, brown, green or black Missing teeth or parts of teeth
Tongue	Pink and moist No coating Visible papillae	Dry Red, white, or black coating Fissures, lesions, swellings
Soft and hard palate	Pink and moist Whiter hard palate	Dry or cracked Red Presence of pus or excessive mucus
Gums	Pink and firm	Redness, inflammation, bleeding Swelling Loose teeth
Saliva	Clear or white Thin Free from odour	Green, brown, yellow or bloodstained Offensive smell
Mucous membrane	Pink, moist, and intact	Pale, red, or discoloured Dry Presence of lesions

Table 60.2 Common oral disorders.

Oral disorders	Signs/symptoms
Xerostomia	Dry mouth
Stomatitis	Inflammation and signs of infection in oral mucosa
Candidiasis	White layer on the tongue and oral mucosa
Gingivitis	Visible swollen gums, usually with redness and bleeding
Ulceration	White, small, lesions

Figure 60.2 Using jug to rinse from the forehead.

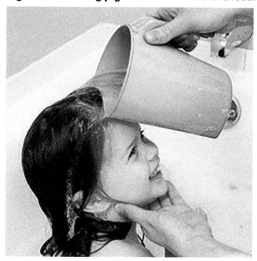

Figure 60.3 Supporting shaving.

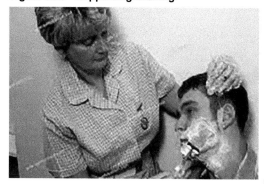

Figure 60.1 Safe position of bed rinser: (a) bed; (b) sink.

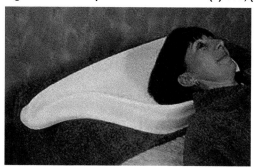
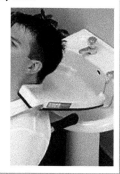

Clinical Nursing Skills at a Glance, First Edition. Edited by Sarah Curr and Carol Fordham-Clarke.
© 2022 John Wiley & Sons Ltd. Published 2022 by John Wiley & Sons Ltd.
Companion website: www.wiley.com/go/clinicalnursingskills

Background

Personal hygiene is not just the cleansing of the body, but also mouth and hair care, including shaving. As all these activities fall under personal care and are performed independently in the well individual, it is important to recognise this and be sensitive as the patient adjusts to requiring support. It is important to support the patient to be as independent as they can while also recognising when they need support with activities.

Influencing Factors

There are many factors that can impact on a person's ability to self-care. These can largely be covered under:

- Individual preference.
- Normal routine.
- Religious traditions.
- Cultural factors.
- Physiological state.
- Psychological state.
- Age.

Professional Approach

- Consider all the above influencing factors and discuss personal preferences as well as what they have been able to do independently while receiving care.
- Ensure that this conversation takes place every time mouth and hair care is delivered, as an individual's ability to self-care will vary.

Equipment

Depending on personal preference equipment could include:

- Toothbrush, toothpaste, mouthwash.
- Small bowl and glass of water.
- Denture tablets and denture pot.
- Bed hair rinser and jug.
- Shampoo, conditioner or equivalent, and hairbrush.
- Razor – patient's own or disposable.
- Face cloth or dry wipes, moisturiser.
- Single-use disposable apron/s and non-sterile gloves.

Procedure – Oral Hygiene

Consider the person's oral hygiene preferences and, where possible, support these. This may involve moving them to a sink to complete their oral hygiene or providing a small bowl and glass of water. If providing oral hygiene, don non-sterile gloves and apron and then assess:

- Lips, teeth, and tongue.
- Mucous membranes and gums.
- Hard and soft palates.
- Saliva production.
- Note any abnormalities (Table 60.1).

As the aim of oral care is to:

- Keep the mucosa clean, soft, moist, and intact.
- Keep the lips clean, soft, moist, and intact.
- Remove food debris and dental plaque.
- Alleviate pain and promote comfort.

- Prevent complications such as infections.
- Promote patient dignity and well-being (Richards and Edwards 2018).

After a full mouth assessment has been performed:

- Cleanse each tooth using either an electric or manual toothbrush.[1] This method will help to ensure that food, debris, and plaque are removed. A mouthwash may also be required.
- Encourage the patient to rinse with water once tooth cleaning is complete.
- For those without teeth, a mouthwash should be used; chlorhexidine is often recommended.
- For those with dentures, ensure that these are soaked overnight in a denture pot. Clean with a soft toothbrush and rinse prior to placement.
- Document care provided and any areas of concern or signs of infection. For common oral disorders signs and symptoms, see Table 60.2.
- Escalate as appropriate – this may require referral to a dentist.

Procedure – Hair Care

- Check what support the person requires, how they usually perform this, and what equipment they require.
- If the patient is mobile take them to the bathroom to cleanse and rinse the hair.
- If the patient is immobile a bed rinser is recommended and, if not available, a large bowl should be used.
- Place the patient into a safe position (Figure 60.1).
- Provide cleansing and rinsing as per patient personal preference, using the jug to rinse from the hairline down (Figure 60.2).
- Remove excess with a towel and use drying devices as available and in accordance with local policy.
- Brush and style hair to patient preference.

Procedure– Shaving

- Ask the patient if they prefer a dry or wet shave (this may be limited by local policy).
- For a wet shave, decontaminate hands and apply apron and non-sterile gloves.
- Wet the face cloth or dry wipes with warm water and apply to the face and neck.
- Apply shaving cream as required.
- Using a safety razor, shave each cheek and moustache in the direction of hair growth, cleansing the razor and the skin after each shave (Figure 60.3).
- Shave the neck using the same method.
- Rinse off excess hair and apply moisturiser as required.
- Document all actions.

Red Flags

☛ Poor oral hygiene can result in local infections which can then travel to the lungs, causing complications such as pneumonia.

References

Richards, A. and Edwards, S.E. (2018). *A Nurse's Survival Guide to the Ward*, 3e. London: Elsevier.

---

1 In gum disease a soft toothbrush may be required.

61 Pressure ulcer – prevention and management

Figure 61.1   Common locations of pressure ulcers. *Source:* Redrawn from C. Lymn.

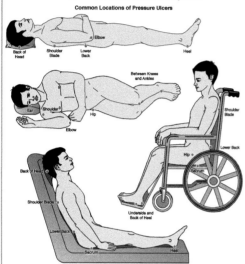

Common Locations of Pressure Ulcers

Table 61.2 Interventions to prevent pressure ulcers.

Intervention	Rationale
Keep skin clean and dry: • pH balanced soap • Barrier cream • Moisturiser • Do not rub • Reduce sweating	Maintain skin integrity Avoid excessive moisture as this exacerbates risk of pressure damage Rehydrate dry skin to reduce risk of damage Rubbing causes friction Avoid heating devices, e.g. hot water bottles, heating pads
Use foam dressings over bony prominences, e.g. heel, sacrum	Provide protection from friction and shear forces Assess skin regularly under dressings and replace if damaged, displaced, or moist
Improve nutritional status and monitor for dehydration	Undertake nutritional screen. If at risk of poor nutrition and hydration, refer to dietician/specialist nurse for individualised nutrition plan Consider use of fortified foods and high-calorie/high-protein supplements
Reposition using turning chart: • Alternate side, back and prone positions • Use moving and handling devices • 30° tilted side-lying position • Head of bed at 30° if on back • Limit time in chair if no pressure relief • Adjust seat position, support feet and arms	Redistribute body weight regularly, improving comfort and hygiene Avoid friction and shear Avoid excess pressure on bony prominences when lying 90° on side Semi-recumbent/slouched positions prone to friction and shear forces Sitting improves mobility but limit to 60 minutes/three times daily if skin damage is evident Maintain position and pressure redistribution; avoid sliding forwards
Use of specialised mattress/bed and support surfaces	If patient is at high risk of developing pressure ulcers and unable to be easily repositioned Refer to tissue viability nurses for implementation and training on use
Keep heels clear of surface if at risk of pressure damage	Position pillow under calves with knee flexed at 10°

Table 61.1 International National Pressure Ulcer Advisory Panel/European Pressure Ulcer Advisory Panel pressure ulcer classification.

Stage	Classification	Description	Picture
Stage I	Non-blanchable erythema	Intact skin with a localised area of non-blanchable redness. May be painful, firmer, softer, warmer, or cooler than surrounding tissue. Detectable in darker skin by heat and colour difference from surrounding tissue	
Stage II	Partial-thickness skin loss	Shallow shiny/dry open ulcer due to loss of dermis; red/pink wound bed with no slough. May also present as serum filled blister	
Stage III	Full-thickness skin loss	Subcutaneous tissue may be visible. Depth dependent upon location	
Stage IV	Full-thickness tissue loss	Bone, tendon, and muscle exposed. Depth dependent upon location. Slough or eschar may be present	
Unstageable	Depth unknown	Stage not evident until slough and/or eschar covering wound bed is removed	

Clinical Nursing Skills at a Glance, First Edition. Edited by Sarah Curr and Carol Fordham-Clarke.
© 2022 John Wiley & Sons Ltd. Published 2022 by John Wiley & Sons Ltd.
Companion website: www.wiley.com/go/clinicalnursingskills

Background

A pressure ulcer is a localised injury to the skin and/or underlying tissue usually over a bony prominence, because of pressure, or pressure and shearing forces (NPUAP/EPUAP/PPPIA 2014). Due to the pressure and injury, perfusion and oxygenation are compromised, resulting in infection and tissue death.

Pressure areas will vary depending on the sitting or lying position of the person (Figure 61.1). As such the patient's usual positions will need to be noted for potential risks to be considered and mitigated against.

Influencing Factors

There are many factors that can place a person at increased risk of developing a pressure ulcer. As such a pressure ulcer risk assessment should be undertaken within six hours of admitting a new patient to any care setting (NICE 2015). The following influencing factors should be considered:

- Reduced mobility.
- Skin condition.
- Perfusion and oxygenation.
- Malnutrition and dehydration.
- Skin moisture, sweat, incontinence.
- Age.
- Neurological impairment.
- Acute/chronic illness.
- Medication.

Professional Approach

- Advise the patient why you are assessing the skin and what you are looking for. The patient can also be advised what to look for and encouraged to report any new onset of pain, numbness, or skin discoloration.

Equipment

Structured risk assessment tools and clinical judgement should be used to assess patients at risk of developing pressure ulcers. Examples include:

- Waterlow scale.
- Braden scale.
- Norton scale.

A pressure ulcer classification tool should also be used when grading a pressure ulcer. This will commonly be the European Pressure Ulcer Advisory Panel (EPUAP) five-stage grading tool (Table 61.1)

Procedure – Preventing Pressure Ulcer Development

In order to prevent pressure development, the above risk assessment tools should be used, in accordance with local policy. For those identified at high risk, the RISE mnemonic (EPUAP 2014) for pressure ulcer prevention can also be implemented:

- **R**eposition.
- **I**nspect.
- **S**kin care.
- **E**at well.

Further details on preventing pressure ulcers can be found in Table 61.2.

Procedure – Skin Assessment

As highlighted in the RISE mnemonic, regular skin inspection is encouraged in all individuals at risk of developing pressure ulcers. This skin assessment should be undertaken:

- Either on initial attendance or within six hours of admission to any care setting.
- When visiting a patient at home.
- With every risk assessment.
- If the patient's condition changes.
- Prior to discharge or transfer to another setting.

The skin assessment should include:

- Performing the blanching response on red areas of skin (see below).
- Checking for:
- localised heat.
- oedema.
- induration/hardness.
- localised discomfort/pain.

Procedure – Assessing the Blanching Response

- *Finger pressure method* – press a finger on the erythema for three seconds. Assess for blanching following removal of finger.
- *Transparent disc method* – apply pressure over the erythema with a transparent disc. Assess for blanching underneath the disc.

Procedure – Pressure Ulcer Classification and Management

Once a pressure ulcer is suspected, either the classification from the EPUAP shown in Table 61.1 or a local care setting validated tool should be used:

- Document the size and depth of the ulcer (NICE 2014) on a wound care chart.
- Document dressing type to be used, when dressing should be changed, and when wound care plan should be reviewed.
- Ensure the appropriate foam mattress is in use.
- Adjust repositioning regime as required.

Red Flags

- ☛ Localised heat, oedema, and induration/hardness are important indicators of pressure damage in patients with darker skin.
- ☛ Assess the skin under and around medical devices (e.g. venous access devices, nasogastric tubes) at least twice daily for signs of pressure damage.

References

European Pressure Ulcer Advisory Panel (EPUAP) (2014) *Preventing Pressure Ulcers*. RISE. https://www.epuap.org/wp-content/uploads/2014/11/RISE-LEaflet-07.05.14-Final-Version.pdf (accessed 1 November 2020).

National Institute of Health and Care Excellence (2014). *CG179 Pressure Ulcers Prevention and Management*. London: National Institute of Health and Care Excellence.

National Institute of Health and Care Excellence (2015). *Q589: Pressure Ulcers*. London: National Institute of Health and Care Excellence.

National Pressure Ulcer Advisory Panel, European Pressure Ulcer Advisory Panel and Pan Pacific Pressure Injury Alliance. (2014) *Prevention and Treatment of Pressure Ulcers: Quick Reference Guide*. (ed. E. Haesler). Osborne Park, Western Australia: Cambridge Media. https://www.epuap.org/wp-content/uploads/2016/10/quick-reference-guide-digital-npuap-epuap-pppia-jan2016.pdf (accessed 25 May 2021).

62 Venous ulcer assessment

Figure 62.1 Skin breakdown and ulcer formation.

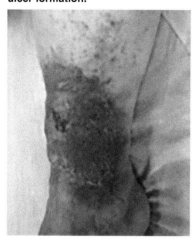

Table 62.1 Assessment of the ulcer.

Ulcer appearance	Observation of the leg
Depth	Oedema
Degree of granulation	Irritation
or epithelialisation	Eczema
Slough	Hyperkeratotic skin
Necrosis	Maceration
Purulence	Cellulitis
Odour	Lipodermatosclerosis
Unusual wound edges	Varicose veins
(e.g. rolled)	Hyperpigmentation
	Atrophie blanche

Source: Based on Regmi and Regmi (2012).

Table 62.2 Venous ulcer assessment.

Ulcer history
Year ulcer first appeared
Site of the ulcer
History of previous ulceration (including number of episodes and time to healing)
Past treatment methods
Previous surgery on venous system
Previous use of compression hosiery or bandaging

Source: Based on Regmi and Regmi (2012).

Figure 62.3 Compression therapy.

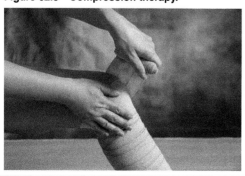

Table 62.3 Physical characteristics of venous ulceration.

Sign	Cause
Absent pedal pulses	Possible peripheral artery disease
Oedema	Plasma proteins and water are lost from the capillaries to the tissues due to pressure changes in the veins
Haemosiderin staining (brown pigmentation of the skin)	Degradation of red blood cells within the epidermis and dermis due to chronic venous disease
Varicose eczema	Irritation of tissues by breakdown products of blood
Lipodermatosclerosis – characterised by hyperpigmented indurated depression of the skin encircling the lower third of both legs, giving the appearance of an inverted bottle	Subcutaneous fibrosis and hardening of the skin on the lower legs due to venous insufficiency
Atrophie blanche – small smooth ivory-white areas on the skin with hyperpigmented borders	Delayed healing following trauma due to venous insufficiency

Source: Adapted from McMonagle and Stephenson (2014).

Figure 62.2 Ankle-brachial pressure index (ABPI) measurement. (a) Treadmill machine for measuring ABPIs before and after exercise. (b) Equipment for measuring ABPI including hand-help Doppler device, BP cuff and manometer and ultrasound gel. (c) Measuring ABPIs at dorsalis pedis artery. Note BP cuff around calf. (d) Typical state-of-the-art vascular ultrasound machine.

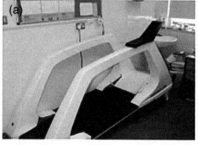
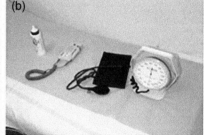
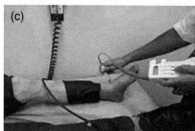
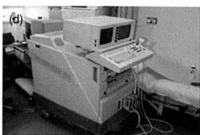

Clinical Nursing Skills at a Glance, First Edition. Edited by Sarah Curr and Carol Fordham-Clarke.
© 2022 John Wiley & Sons Ltd. Published 2022 by John Wiley & Sons Ltd.
Companion website: www.wiley.com/go/clinicalnursingskills

Background

Venous Ulceration

Venous ulceration presents as a chronic wound, mostly along the medial distal lower limb, which occurs due to dysfunction of the venous system (McMonagle and Stephenson 2014). This ulceration occurs when there is damage to any of the three systems of veins that exist in the lower limbs: the superficial, deep, and perforating veins.

This damage could be as a result of any of the following three mechanisms failing:

- The action of the calf muscle pump which forces blood in the deep veins forward.
- Pouch-like valves which open towards the heart, thereby preventing back flow.
- Pressure variations within the abdomen and thorax.

The high venous pressure and backflow cause chronic venous hypertension (Regmi and Regmi 2012). The resulting chronic oedema leads to increased capillary permeability with subsequent tissue ischaemia, resulting in skin breakdown and the formation of the ulcer (Figure 62.1).

Arterial Aetiology

Ulcers on the lower limb may also result from arterial dysfunction, most often due to atherosclerotic disease – causing arterial stenosis and tissue ischaemia. As such it is imperative that any arterial involvement is excluded prior to commencing leg ulcer treatment (McMonagle and Stephenson 2014). A mixed aetiology may also present in patients with ulceration development who have coexistent arterial disease; these often appear suddenly and deteriorate rapidly. Likewise, arterial disease can develop in a patient with long-standing venous ulceration.

In patients with diabetes ulceration, there may be micro-and macrovascular changes in the blood vessels in combination with peripheral neuropathy. This is associated with tissue breakdown and poor healing, and thus all patients presenting with an ulcer must be screened for arterial disease.

Influencing Factors

- Venous disease.
- Arterial disease.
- Venous thrombosis.
- Diabetes mellitus.
- Rheumatoid arthritis.

Professional Approach

- Ensure that you explain what you will be doing in all aspects of your assessment and why.
- Provide health education and information on optimal leg ulcer management.
- Provide details of standard time-frame for healing (12 weeks).

Procedure – Assessment

A detailed patient assessment is essential in venous ulceration and should include:

- A full clinical history including ulcer and past medical history.
- A physical examination to identify any comorbidities (Regmi and Regmi 2012) (Tables 62.1 and 62.2).
- A physical assessment to identify any characteristics of venous disease (Table 62.3).
- A swab for microbiological investigation – if there is evidence of pyrexia, inflammation, redness, cellulitis or purulent exudate.[1]

Procedure – Ankle-Brachial Pressure Index (ABPI) Measurement (Figure 62.2)

- This is the ratio of the blood pressure in the legs to the blood pressure in the arms and should be performed on anyone presenting with tissue breakdown and ulceration.
- The ankle-brachial pressure index (ABPI) should then be assessed every three months, and also when an ulcer is deteriorating or when it is not fully healed by 12 weeks.
- A sudden increase in pain or ulcer size, or a change in foot colour or warmth should also prompt an ABPI check.

NB: ABPI measurement and pedal pulse assessment should only be carried out by a trained healthcare professional.

Leg Ulcer Management

The aims of management are to improve quality of life, reduce pain, correct underlying causes, and create an optimum environment for wound healing. The key treatment is:

- Graduated compression therapy via the application of elasticated bandages applied by a competent healthcare practitioner (Figure 62.3) (Regmi and Regmi 2012).
- Patient education, which should include information on leg elevation, exercise, and compliance with compression.

Red Flags

- Absence of pedal pulses.
- Non-healing ulcer despite treatment.

References

McMonagle, M. and Stephenson, M. (2014). *Vascular and Endovascular Surgery at a Glance*. Oxford: Wiley.
Regmi, S. and Regmi, K. (2012). Best practice in the management of venous leg ulcers. *Nursing Standard* 26 (32): 56–66.

---

1 Rapid deterioration of the ulcer can also be a sign of infection, as can increased pain from the ulcer.

63 Wound dressing using aseptic non-touch technique (ANTT)

Figure 63.1   Check for expiry dates.

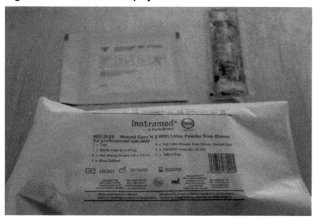

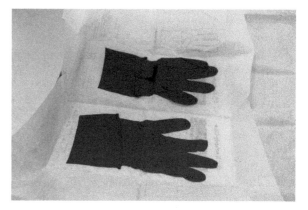

Figure 63.2   Sterile field.

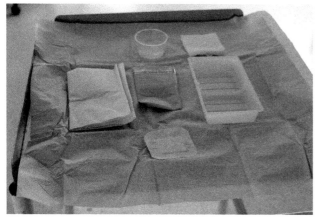

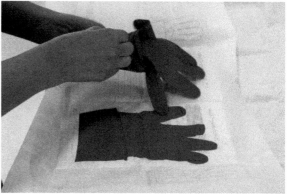

Figure 63.3   Putting <u>on</u> sterile gloves.

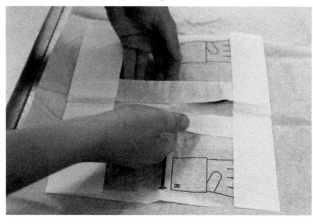

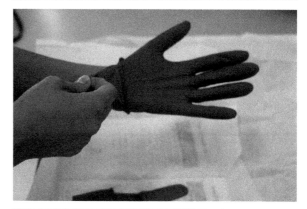

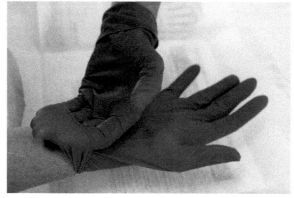

Background

The use of an aseptic non-touch technique (ANTT) is an important infection control procedure. Asepsis refers to the state of being free of pathogenic microorganisms which may cause localised infection, poor wound healing, patient deterioration, sepsis, and life-threatening illness (ASAP 2015). Any intervention which bypasses the body's natural defences of the skin or mucous membranes and enables possible contamination by microorganisms may cause infection. An ANTT should be used when undertaking any invasive procedure such as venepuncture and urinary catheter insertion (Loveday et al. 2014). The following information relates specifically to wound care.

Influencing Factors

- Those providing ANTT must be trained in this approach and follow local policy.
- Prior to the procedure, consider patient-influencing factors such as pain and mobility but also scheduled visitors and procedures.

Professional approach.

- Ensure that informed consent is obtained.
- Consider privacy and dignity.
- Follow the wound care plan.

Equipment

Equipment used will depend upon the procedure undertaken but will include the following:

- Chlorhexidine hard surface cleansing wipes 70% alcohol or recommendation of local Trust policy.
- Dressing pack containing gauze, gallipot, waste bag.
- Sterile gloves.
- Personal protective equipment (PPE).
- Cleansing solution.
- Wound dressing.
- Alcohol-based hand decontamination gel.

  Additional items may include:

- Sterile scissors or forceps.
- Additional PPE such as a mask or goggles.
- Extra gauze.
- 10 mL sterile syringe for irrigation.

Procedure

There may be variations in ANTT procedures, but the following principles must be applied at all times (Aziz 2009):

- Rigorous hand hygiene.
- A non-touch technique.
- Reduced risk of airborne cross-contamination.
- Use of sterile equipment, including gloves and cleansing solutions (Loveday et al. 2014).

In the clinical environment, a clean dressing trolley free of visible contamination will be used, both for the transport of equipment and as a clean work surface. In a community setting, a clean flat surface should be selected, such as a table, and cleaned as much as possible.

Procedure – Redressing a Wound using ANTT

- Explain procedure and obtain verbal consent.
- Ensure patient comfort, adjusting bedclothes as necessary.
- Check allergy status and wound care plan.
- Decontaminate hands.
- Clean the dressing trolley using chlorhexidine in 70% alcohol or as per local policy.
- Gather equipment on the bottom shelf of the trolley checking expiry dates and integrity of packaging or autoclave tape (Figure 63.1).
- Take trolley to patient and close curtains/door to maintain privacy.
- Decontaminate hands and put on disposable apron.
- Loosen the dressing and decontaminate hands.
- Remove the dressing pack from outer packaging and slide onto the top of the dressing trolley.
- Open the pack, touching only the corners of the paper to create a sterile field.
- Open items required and place onto the sterile field, including pouring the cleansing solution into the gallipot using a non-touch technique (Figure 63.2).
- Decontaminate hands.
- Pick up the waste bag and, placing a hand inside like a glove, rearrange items on the sterile field.
- With the hand in the waste bag, remove the soiled dressing, invert the bag with the dressing enclosed, and attach to the side of the trolley next to the patient.
- Put on sterile gloves, avoiding contamination (Figure 63.3).
- Open the dressing towel and place close to the wound.
- Moisten gauze swab in cleansing solution and clean wound, from clean to dirty areas, using each swab only once.
- Alternatively, irrigate wound using a syringe from a height of 5 cm above the wound.
- Use gauze to dry around the wound, again using each swab only once.
- Apply dressing – press gently to ensure adherence.
- Remove dressing towel, wrap all items in the sterile field, and place in a waste bag.
- Remove gloves and place in the waste bag, detaching it from the trolley.
- Dispose of waste in clinical waste bin and decontaminate hands.
- Check patient and ensure comfort before leaving.
- Clean trolley as per local policy and attach green decontamination label.

Procedure – Clean Technique

In some situations, it is permissible to use a "clean technique". This is similar to the aseptic technique, but the use of sterile equipment is not required: e.g. when dressing a chronic wound such as venous ulceration. Remember that factors such as patient's level of immunity, age, and nutritional status must be considered. If in doubt an aseptic technique should be performed.

Red Flags

- ☛ Provide analgesia if required prior to procedure.
- ☛ Take appropriately sized sterile gloves if those in the dressing pack are not the correct size.
- ☛ Maintain integrity of sterile field throughout and ensure key parts are not contaminated.

References

Aziz, A.M. (2009). Variations in aseptic technique and implications for infection control. *British Journal of Nursing* 18 (1): 26–31.

Loveday, H., Wilson, J.A., Pratt, R. et al. (2014). epic3: National Evidence-Based Guidelines for preventing healthcare-associated infections in NHS hospitals in England. *Journal of Hospital Infection* 86: S1–S70.

Association for Safe Aseptic Practice (2015). *Aseptic Non-Touch Technique*. London: Association for Safe Aseptic Practice.

64 Burns management

Table 64.1 Burn types and characteristics.

Burn type	Area affected	Characteristics
Epidermal burn	Skin	Red, dry, no blisters, painful
Superficial partial-thickness burn	Epidermis, part of papillary dermis	Red, blisters, swelling, painful
Deep partial-thickness burn	Epidermis, entire papillary dermis, reticular dermis	White, may look leathery, no pain
Full-thickness burn	Entire thickness of skin, potentially subcutaneous tissue (requires surgery)	Charred, eschar

Figure 64.1 Lund and Bowder chart.

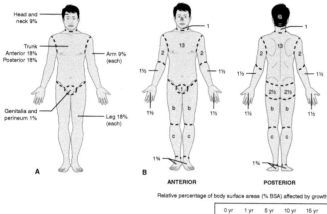

Figure 64.2 Wallace rule of nines for adults.

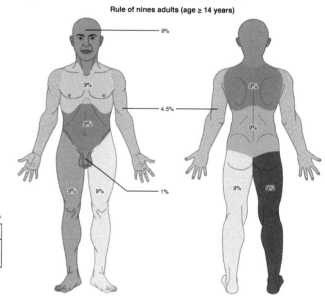

Table 64.2 A–E assessment in burns injuries.

Assessment	Additional in burns injuries
Airway	Signs of swelling of airway, i.e. stridor
Breathing	Signs of inhalation injury, i.e. dark mucus, cough
Circulation	Consider fluid replacement requirements, specifically in adults with over 15% total body surface area (TBSA), 10% TBSA in the elderly
Disability	Signs of hypothermia, neurovascular assessment, i.e. signs of compartment syndrome
Exposure	Percentage of burn area affected

Clinical Nursing Skills at a Glance, First Edition. Edited by Sarah Curr and Carol Fordham-Clarke.
© 2022 John Wiley & Sons Ltd. Published 2022 by John Wiley & Sons Ltd.
Companion website: www.wiley.com/go/clinicalnursingskills

Background

Burns are a recognised global problem due to frequency of occurrence, preventable incidences of mortality, and the long-term physical and psychological effects (WHO 2018). As such, timely, effective treatment is required, and the healthcare professional must have the knowledge and skill to provide this. To be able to treat people with burn injuries in all care settings, the healthcare professional must be aware of the four main types of burn:

- Thermal.
- Chemical.
- Electric.
- Radiation.

The healthcare professional must also understand the physiology of the skin and recognise the different burn categories, classified as:

- Epidermal.
- Superficial partial thickness.
- Deep partial thickness.
- Full thickness (Table 64.1).

This underlying knowledge, combined with practical experience to build competency, will enable the healthcare professional to provide initial first aid, pain management, detailed assessment, and dressing of the wound. An awareness of when to escalate care is also of fundamental importance here.

Influencing Factors

Whilst superficial burns will heal without much intervention, partial burns require pain management, dressings and ongoing care and some burns warrant referral to a specialist burn centre. These are:

- All full thickness burns.
- All circumference burns.
- All burns that are more than 2% in children, (Figure 64.1), and more than 3% in adults (Figure 64.2).
- Significant burns to hands, feet, face, perineum, genitalia.
- Cold injuries.
- Chemical, friction or electrical burns (NNBC 2012).

Professional Approach

Whilst not all patients with a burn will present with pain all patients will require immediate and sensitive treatment. It is essential to ascertain if the injury was accidental/non-accidental and escalate to the appropriate services, as necessary. Immediate care will impact on the long-term result and thus acting quickly may be of paramount concern. Despite this it is essential to reassure the patient by explaining each part of the process so that they are aware of what is happening and why.

Equipment

Non-sterile gloves.
Disposable apron.
Burn assessment chart (Figures 64.1 and 64.2).
Fresh running water (first aid).
Appropriate dressing.
Wound care pack.
Sterile gloves.
Cleansing agent i.e. 0.9% sodium chloride.

Procedure – Immediate First Aid

Depending on the type of burn you will need to stop the burning by removing the cause of the burn. Then follow the below steps:

- Remove clothing and or jewellery.
- Cool the burn for up to 30 minutes.
- Perform an A–E assessment (Table 64.2).
- Cover the burn (PVC such as clingfilm but laid over the burn, not wrapped).
- Pain management (paracetamol, low to moderate opioid ± non-steroid anti-inflammatory) (Wounds International 2014).

Procedure – Assessment

Once immediate first aid and analgesia has been provided take a full history of the burn including mechanism of injury and time it occurred. Ascertain:

- The burn category.
- The size using the appropriate chart (Figure 65.1 and 65.2) remembering to not count epidermal burns.
- Try to gauge burn depth.

This will help ascertain if referral to a specialist centre is required, if intravenous therapy is needed, and help you consider what type of dressing to provide.

Procedure – Wound Dressing

Dressings are only required for superficial partial and deep partial thickness burns. Epidermal burns do not require a dressing and full thickness burns require surgery and transfer to a specialist burn centre. When considering the dressing consider:

- Exudate – if high exudate use a foam dressing, for low exudate a film dressing.
- Signs of infection - use a silver or honey impregnated dressing.

Ensure that the dressing:

- Creates a moist wound environment.
- Retains close contact with the wound bed.
- Contours easily.
- Is painless on both application and removal (Carta et al. 2018).

For all dressing applications and removal, follow the aseptic non-touch procedure outlined in Chapter 63. Dressings should be changed:

- Within the first 48 hours.
- Every three to five days.
- If painful or malodorous.

NB: If signs of infection swab and send for microscopic culture and sensitivity.

Red Flag

- Non-accidental injury.
- A transparent film, with cellophane base, can make a chemical burn worse.
- Do not irrigate electrical burns.
- Do not use ice or cold water when providing initial first aid as this can further damage the wound.

References

Carta, T., Gawaziwk, J.P., Diaz-Abele, J. et al. (2018). Properties of an ideal burn dressing: a survey of burn survivors and front-line burn healthcare providers. *Burns* 45 (2019): 364–368.
National Network for Burns Care (NNBC) (2012) *National Burn Care Referral Guidance.* https://www.britishburnassociation.org/wp-content/uploads/2018/02/National-Burn-Care-Referral-Guidance-2012.pdf (accessed 25 November 2020).
World Health Organization (2018) *Violence and Injury Prevention: Burns.* https://www.who.int/violence_injury_prevention/other_injury/burns/en (accessed 25 November 2020).
Wounds International (2014). *International Best Practice Guidelines: Effective Skin and Wound Management of Non-complex Burns.* London: Wound International.

65 **Care after death**

Table 65.1 Causes of death to be reported to Coroner.

A doctor did not treat the person during the period of illness

A doctor did not see or treat the person within 28 days of death

There is a question of negligence

Death was due to poisoning

Death was due to exposure to a toxic substance (medical or non-medical)

Cause of death was murder

Cause of death was a violent act, i.e. accident

Cause of death was a result of self-harm

Cause of death classified as unnatural

The person cannot be identified

Figure 65.2 Body bag.

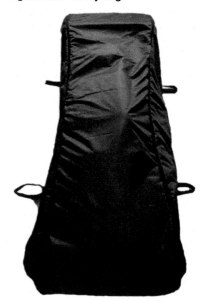

Figure 65.1 Loosely wrap the patient in a sheet.

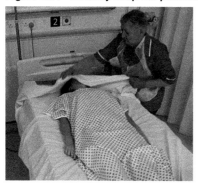
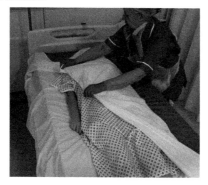
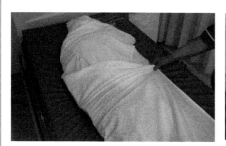
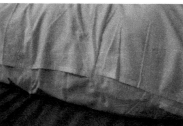

Figure 65.3 Cause of Death certificate.

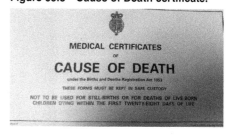
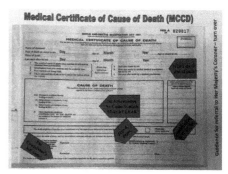

Clinical Nursing Skills at a Glance, First Edition. Edited by Sarah Curr and Carol Fordham-Clarke.
© 2022 John Wiley & Sons Ltd. Published 2022 by John Wiley & Sons Ltd.
Companion website: www.wiley.com/go/clinicalnursingskills

Background

- The physical preparation of the body after death, traditionally referred to as "last offices", involves the personal care of the patient from the time of death to collection by the hospital porters or the funeral directors.
- Care after death also includes, where possible, the cultural, religious, and personal preferences of the deceased and those close to them, within legal obligations (NHSE 2017).

Influencing Factors

- Before commencing the care after death procedure, verification of death must be obtained from a doctor or approved nurse with confirmation written in the patient notes as per national and local guidance (Ministry of Justice 2020).
- Personal protective equipment (PPE) must be worn – as a minimum, non-sterile gloves and aprons.
- Safe moving and handling guidance must be followed with two people representing best practice.
- Care after death may also include preparing the deceased for viewing where appropriate and the support of family/friends with this.
- Care after death includes following a person's wishes for organ, tissue, and whole-body donation.
- Legal requirements must be met if a death is to be reported to the Coroner (Table 65.1), a postmortem is required, or a safeguarding issue becomes evident after death.
- If the person had a known or suspected infection, local infection control policy must also be followed including reporting to necessary personnel and agencies.

Professional Approach

- The privacy and dignity of the deceased person must always be maintained, and the surrounding environment should convey the necessary respect.
- Empathic and clear communication is required, tailoring information to the needs of family and carers, including informing those not present at the time of death.
- Family members and/or carers should be allowed to sit with the deceased immediately after death. They may wish to participate in the care of the deceased and should be supported to do so if they wish.
- Record all aspects of care after death in nursing and medical documentation and identify the professionals involved.

Equipment

- PPE.
- Washing items (Chapter 59).
- Mouth care items (Chapter 60).
- Brush or comb.
- Shaving equipment (Chapter 60).
- Shroud or clean nightwear.
- Clean bed sheet.
- Adhesive tape.
- Continence pads and body bag if required.
- Name bands.

Procedure

- Move the deceased onto their back, head supported by a pillow, and limbs straightened, if possible, with the arms at their sides.
- Support the jaw with a pillow or rolled-up towel and remove before viewing.
- Clean the mouth of debris and secretions – this includes cleaning and replacing dentures.
- Tidy the hair into the preferred style.
- Apply light pressure for 30 seconds to close the eyes, if possible.
- Remove jewellery, apart from a wedding ring, in the presence of another staff member and document as per local policy. Any rings left on the deceased should be secured with tape.
- Cover all wounds with a waterproof absorbent dressing then secure with an occlusive dressing, leaving stitches or clips intact. Indwelling devices stay in situ, capped off, clamped or spigotted as appropriate (Hospice 2015).
- If the case is to be referred to the coroner then advice should be sought before moving or removing anything from the body.
- Invasive lines must be left in situ, drains clamped and the bottle removed, and urinary catheter spigotted. Local policy must be followed.
- The deceased should be washed, unless cultural or religious requests have been otherwise made from family members/carers.
- If leakage is not expected, the deceased may be placed into a disposable shroud or their own clean nightwear and then loosely wrapped in a clean sheet which is taped lightly (Figure 65.1).
- If leakage from any orifice occurs, or is expected, insert gauze packing, following local policy. Place the deceased on absorbent pads in a body (cadaver) bag and advise the mortuary or funeral director (HSE 2018).
- If there are infection control issues the deceased may be placed into a body bag (Figure 65.2).
- Attach identification labels to the body as per local guidelines.
- A Cause of Death certificate (Figure 65.3) must be completed and attached to the patient's medical records (Ministry of Justice 2020).
- Personal property should be packed with sensitivity for the feelings of those receiving it in line with local policy.
- Written information should be given to the family members/carers about the processes that take place after death. They should also be supported to view the body after collection if they so wish.

NB: Personal care should be performed within three to four hours of death to preserve dignity, appearance, and condition.

Red Flags

- Shaving can cause delayed bruising and marking – discuss the need with the family first.
- Ensure any sheet or tape is not too tight as this can cause disfigurement.
- Inform mortuary staff about any implanted devices such as a pacemaker or defibrillator (NHS England 2017).

References

Health and Safety Executive (HSE) (2018) *Managing Infection Risks when Handling the Deceased.* www.hse.gov.uk/pubns/priced/hsg283.pdf (accessed 25 November 2020).

Hospice, U.K. (2015). *Care after Death: Guidance for Staff Responsible for Care after Death.* London: Hospice UK.

Ministry of Justice (2020) *Revised Guidance for Registered Medical Practitioners on the Notifications of Death Regulations.* https://assets.publishing.service.gov.uk/government/uploads/system/uploads/attachment_data/file/878083/revised-guidance-for-registered-medical-practitioners-on-the-notification-of-deaths-regulations.pdf (accessed 25 November 2020).

NHS England (2017) *Guidance for Staff Responsible for Care after Death (Last Offices).* National End of Life Care Programme. https://www.england.nhs.uk/improvement-hub/wp-content/uploads/sites/44/2017/10/Guidance-for-Staff-Responsible-for-Care-after-Death.pdf (accessed on 25 May 2021).

66 Management of surgical drains

Table 66.1 Types of surgical drain.

Type of drain	Action
Open	Uses capillarity or gravity to drain into a dressing or stoma bag inserted over the site, e.g. corrugated drain A large sterile safety pin is often placed through the drain outside the insertion site to prevent slippage back through the incised area. Shortening an open drain (drawing back in increments) may be ordered 1–2 days before removal to bring the drain closer to the skin surface to promote healing from the wound base
Closed	Consists of a tube draining into a bag or bottle, e.g. abdominal drains and chest drains
Active	Maintained under suction which uses gentle negative pressure to drain the fluid into a vacuumed device, e.g. Redivac® drain, bulb, or concertina drains
Passive	Has no suction and drainage is by pressure differential, gravity, and overflow, e.g. abdominal drains

Figure 66.2   Closed active drain, with and without vacuum.

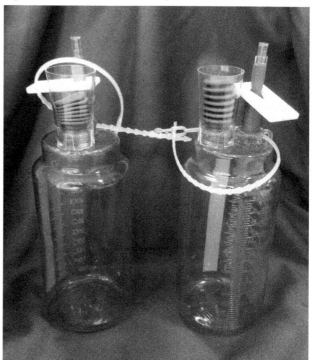

Figure 66.1   Different types of surgical drain.

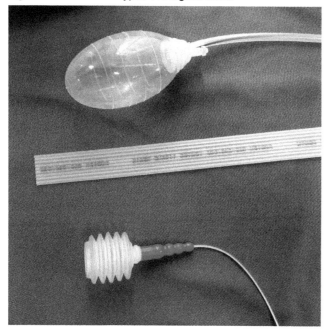

Clinical Nursing Skills at a Glance, First Edition. Edited by Sarah Curr and Carol Fordham-Clarke.
© 2022 John Wiley & Sons Ltd. Published 2022 by John Wiley & Sons Ltd.
Companion website: www.wiley.com/go/clinicalnursingskills

Background

A drain is a tube placed lateral to the surgical incision, exiting the body usually through a separate small opening. The drain is placed in order to:

- Prevent the transmission of infection to the surgical wound.
- Decompress the wound by eliminating dead space and prevent the accumulation of blood, or fluids in the wound bed (Knowlton 2015).
- Form a controlled fistula for the diversion of fluids from the surgical site, e.g. a T-tube drain after common bile duct exploration.

   NB: Any formation of haematoma or fluid accumulation could become a focus of infection or irritate surrounding tissues and potentially lead to wound dehiscence. Volume and type of fluid lost can be monitored facilitating replacement.

Influencing Factors

Draining systems are affected by:

- Surgery undertaken.
- Wound.
- Amount of drainage anticipated.
- Surgeon's preferred technique.
- Being sutured to the skin to prevent dislodgement.

Professional Approach

- Explain why the drain is in situ and what you are looking for when assessing it.
- Encourage the person to inform you of any pain or discomfort at site and to notify you if they notice any other changes.

Procedure – Management of Drains

Depends upon type, purpose, and location (Figure 66.1; Table 66.1).

- All management will involve monitoring and documenting drainage in the patient record:
  - Colour.
  - Consistency.
  - Volume.
- Label multiple drains for clear identification.
- Document drainage volumes, in fluid balance chart, with each set of observations postoperatively, up to a minimum of four-hourly.
- If output increases, increase frequency of monitoring.
- Ensure antennae or bellows on top of bottle in active drains indicate that negative pressure is primed at all times and reinstate if lost (Durai and Ng 2010). (Figure 66.2).
- Ensure drain is located below the level of the insertion site.
- Observe for kinks in the tubing or if it is trapped under the patient.
- If infection is suspected at the drain site, report to the medical team immediately. If discharge is present, take a swab or sample for microbiological investigation.
- Take care when moving a patient with a drain to prevent pain or dislodgement.
- Assess the patient, insertion site, and security of drain both before and after moving the patient.
- If drainage appears minimal or ceases abruptly, ensure drainage tubing is not kinked or blocked. If unable to reinstate patency of drainage system, inform medical team immediately.

Procedure – Dressing a Site

- Following verbal consent, use aseptic technique to remove the drain dressing.
- Assess insertion site for leakage, redness, or signs of infection.
- Clean drain insertion site with 0.9% sodium chloride while assessing the surrounding skin.
- Check drain security. Sutures may be used.
- Use a non-adherent dressing to cover the drain site.
- Document procedure including site condition.

   For an open drain:
- Observe any safety pins used remains visible, secure, and close to the skin.
- Use enough padding to absorb drainage and redress as required to prevent saturation or apply drainage bag over the insertion site.

   If shortening an open drain:
- Follow guidelines above but before re-dressing gently pull the tubing out of the wound by length required (usually 2–5 cm).
- Place sterile safety pin across the tubing at 90° to prevent retraction back into the wound and re-dress.

Procedure – Changing a Closed Active Drainage System

Using an aseptic technique:

- Assess volume of drainage in current device and document on fluid chart.
- Close clamp on the drainage tube and clamp on bottle connector.
- Disconnect bottle from tubing, ensuring the end of drainage tubing is not touched.
- Clean the end of tubing and attach a new sterile drainage device.
- Ensure both clamps are unclamped and the vacuum indicator on the bottle signals negative pressure.
- Leaving clamp in situ on used bottle, dispose of it into the clinical waste bag (Figure 66.2).

Procedure – Removing a Closed Drain

A drain should stay in situ for the minimum length of time required to reduce the risk of infection or mechanical damage which also reduces the risk of granulation around the drain, minimising trauma and reducing pain on removal. Removal occurs following medical advice and when drainage has decreased sufficiently, i.e. less than 25–50 mL/24 hours.

   Using an aseptic technique:

- If an active drainage system, remove negative pressure prior to removal (Durai and Ng 2010).
- Remove drain site dressing and clean if necessary to visualise suture.
- Remove any sutures, securing the drain.
- Holding a sterile gauze with a finger on each side of the insertion site, use gentle traction to withdraw the drain. Do not use excessive force. If resistance is met, redress and seek medical advice.
- Apply an absorbent dressing.
- Check and document removal of the complete drain.

Red Flags

- Ensure the patient is aware that the drain should be kept below the level of the wound and understands the necessary care to prevent pain or dislodgement.
- Ensure appropriate analgesia is administered as prescribed, particularly prior to shortening or removal of the drain.
- If the patient is to be discharged home with the drain in place, ensure that sufficient education is given for care of the drain.

References

Durai, R. and Ng, P. (2010). Surgical vacuum drains: types, uses, and complications. *AORN Journal* 91 (2): 266–274.
Knowlton, M.C. (2015). Nurse's guide to surgical drain removal. *Nursing* 45 (9): 59–61.

67 Suture and staple removal

Figure 67.1   Suture techniques.

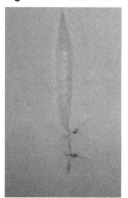 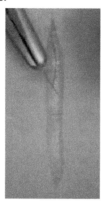 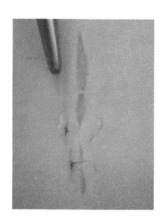 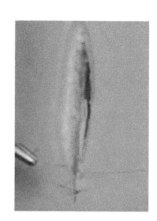

Figure 67.2   Staples.

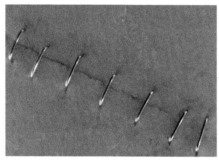

Figure 67.3   Skin adhesive – glue.

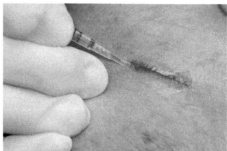

Figure 67.5   Equipment for removal of sutures and staples.

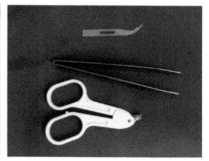

Figure 67.6   Using a stitch cutter.

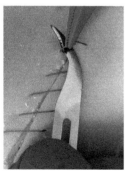

Figure 67.7   Removing staples.

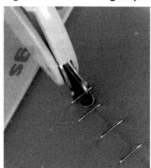

Figure 67.4   Skin adhesive – SteriStrips.

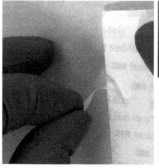 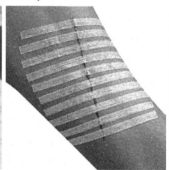

Clinical Nursing Skills at a Glance, First Edition. Edited by Sarah Curr and Carol Fordham-Clarke.
© 2022 John Wiley & Sons Ltd. Published 2022 by John Wiley & Sons Ltd.
Companion website: www.wiley.com/go/clinicalnursingskills

Background

Wound closure after injury or surgery brings together the wound edges to support and strengthen the wound, enabling healing by primary intention, reducing the risk of blood loss and infection. Methods of wound closure will depend upon the type of wound. Commonly used methods of skin closure include:

- Sutures.
- Staples.
- Adhesive strips.
- Tissue adhesive ("liquid stitches" or glue).

Sutures

Suture techniques vary according to wound type and location (Figure 67.1). The suture material may be absorbable or non-absorbable. Absorbable sutures do not require removal, as they will be absorbed over a two-week period.

Staples

Staples are frequently used to close surgical wounds or scalp lacerations (Figure 67.2), as they are quicker and more economical than sutures, causing fewer infections (Armitage and Lockwood 2011).

Skin adhesive ("liquid stitches" or glue)

This is often used for superficial lacerations (Figure 67.3). It forms a film that holds the edges of the wound together and naturally sloughs off in around seven days.

Adhesive wound closure strips ("butterfly /paper stitches" or "SteriStrips")

These can be applied to small, superficial, lacerations instead of sutures to pull the skin together (Reynolds and Cole 2006,) (Figure 67.4), but it is recommended that they are not used for deeper wounds, requiring tension, and the strips will not be able to hold the margins together adequately (Bonham 2016). They may also be applied after suture or staple removal to support the tensile strength of the wound and should be left in situ until they fall off.

Influencing Factors – Types of Skin Closure

Choice of wound closure material will depend on the site of the wound, its size, and depth. Removal occurs when enough tensile strength is established to hold the wound edges together. The timing of suture or staple removal should be carefully considered to reduce the risk of permanent scarring while ensuring sufficient wound strength to prevent dehiscence.

Professional Approach

Obtain informed verbal consent before starting the procedure and answer any questions to relieve anxiety. Follow infection control procedures to prevent wound infection and cross-contamination.

Procedure

- The time-frame for removal of sutures or staples varies according to wound location, usually between 7 and 10 days. Face and neck closures can sometimes be removed at five days due to enhanced vascularity.
- The wound and surrounding skin must be inspected daily prior to suture or staple removal, and prompt referral to the appropriate team is required if wound infection is suspected. This may result in the removal of some or all of the sutures to allow for drainage of infection.

NB: Appropriate analgesia should be administered prior to removal of sutures or staples. Recent research supports using a lidocaine patch (Tseng et al. 2017). Ensure that the patient is assisted into a comfortable position to allow easy access to the wound.

Procedure – Removal of Sutures

1 Assemble and prepare the equipment as for aseptic non-touch technique (ANTT) plus a stitch cutter, sterile adhesive strips, tweezers, or forceps (Figure 67.5).
2 Clean the wound with 0.9% sodium chloride to remove encrusted blood/secretions.
3 When cutting the suture, it is important to prevent infection by ensuring exposed suture material is not pulled through the wound.
4 Grasp the knot of the suture using the forceps, gently raise it off the skin and cut the suture close to the skin using the stitch cutter (Figure 67.6).
5 Avoiding excessive force, pull the suture out towards the side that was cut and gently press the skin close to the wound with your free hand.
6 Remove alternate sutures first and assess wound adherence before continuing to remove all sutures.
7 Inspect the wound to ensure all sutures have been removed and apply a wound dressing.

Procedure – Removal of Staples

1 Assemble the equipment for ANTT plus a staple remover.
2 Slide the lower bar of the staple remover under the staple and squeeze the handles together until the staple is fully open and remove (Figure 67.7).
3 If the wound is under tension, use the free hand to gently squeeze the skin on either side of the wound.
4 Once completed, inspect the wound to ensure all staples have been removed and apply a wound dressing.

NB: Details of suture or staple removal as well as an assessment of the wound and surrounding skin must be documented in the patient record. If the patient is discharged home with skin closure in situ, education about wound care and details of the arrangements made for suture or staple removal must be provided.

Red Flags

- Leaving sutures or staples in situ for too long may lead to excessive scarring.
- If resistance is met when pulling out a suture, use a slow, continuous pulling motion.
- Do not pull exposed suture material through the wound as this could cause contamination.
- Where wound healing is impaired, sutures or staples may be left in situ for longer, e.g. the elderly, malnourished.

References

Armitage, J. and Lockwood, S. (2011). Skin incisions and wound closure. *Surgery* 29 (10): 496–501.

Bonham, J. (2016). Assessment and management of patients with minor traumatic wounds. *Nursing Standard* 31 (8): 60–69.

Reynolds, T. and Cole, E. (2006). Techniques for acute wound closure. *Nursing Standard* 20 (21): 55–64.

Tseng, T.-H., Jiang, C.-C., Fu, S.-H., and Lee, T.-L. (2017). Topical anesthesia for staple removal from surgical wounds on the knee: a prospective, double-blind, randomized trial. *Journal of Surgical Research* 215: 167–172.

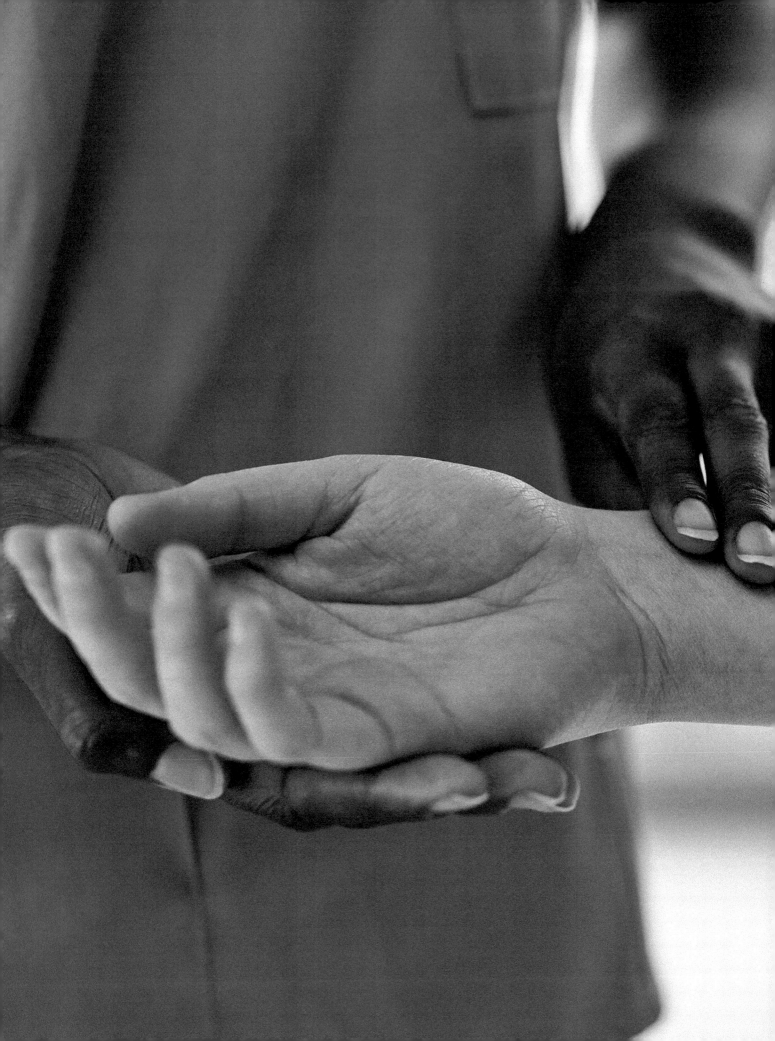

Endocrine skills

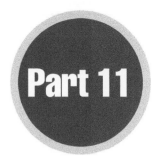

Part 11

Chapter

68 Capillary blood glucose monitoring

Figure 68.1 Effects of insulin and glucagon on blood sugar levels. *Source*: Redrawn from Wallymahmed (2007).

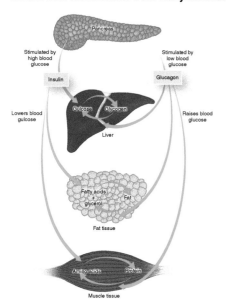

Figure 68.2 Capillary blood glucose equipment.

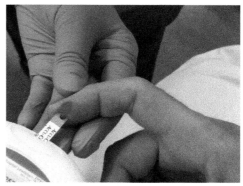

Figure 68.4 Glucose and glycated haemoglobin (HbA1c) levels.

	HbA1c test score	MEAN BLOOD GLUCOSE	
		mg/dL	mmol/L
Diabetes Control Card	14.0	380	21.1
	13.0	350	19.3
	12.0	315	17.4
	11.0	280	15.6
	10.0	250	13.7
	9.0	215	11.9
	8.0	180	10.0
	7.0	150	8.2
	6.0	115	6.3
	5.0	80	4.7
	4.0	50	2.6

Table 68.1 Signs of hypoglycaemia and hyperglycaemia.

Hypoglycaemia	Hyperglycaemia
Sweating	Increased thirst (polydipsia)
Shaking	Increased urine output (polyuria)
Palpitations	Blurred vision
Hunger	Headache
Nausea	Glycosuria
Poor concentration	Fatigue
Blurred vision	Difficulty concentrating
Dizziness	Altered level of consciousness
Anxiety	
Irritability	
Confusion	

Table 68.2 Accuracy of capillary blood glucose.

Conditions that may affect capillary blood glucose result accuracy
Peripheral circulatory failure
Severe dehydration
Haematocrit > 55%
Hyperlipidaemia
High serum bilirubin levels
Intravenous infusion of ascorbic acid
Some renal dialysis treatments

Source: Based on Wallymahmed (2007).

Figure 68.3 Taking a capillary blood glucose.

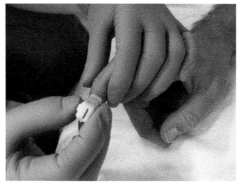

Background

The islets of Langerhans are clusters of cells that secrete the hormones insulin and glucagon directly into the pancreatic veins. They are irregularly distributed throughout the pancreas. These two hormones work together to balance the levels of glucose in the blood (Figure 68.1; Wallymahmed 2007):

- Glucagon is secreted by alpha (α) cells in response to low blood glucose levels, raising the levels of glucose in the blood by releasing glycogen stores from the liver.
- Insulin is secreted by the beta (β) cells, which are stimulated by elevated blood glucose levels.
- Insulin reduces the levels of blood glucose by enabling glucose to enter the cells to be catabolised, thus producing energy and heat while also stimulating the conversion of excess glucose to glycogen for storage in muscle and liver cells.

NB: The production of insufficient amounts of insulin by the pancreas will result in the patient developing the chronic condition diabetes mellitus.

Influencing Factors

Capillary blood glucose may be monitored for numerous reasons (Holt 2014):

- To detect hypoglycaemia or hyperglycaemia, allowing for prompt initiation of appropriate treatment.
- To reduce the risk of developing the acute complications of type 1 and type 2 diabetes.
- To manage diabetic control of patients when this control may be affected by illness, fasting, modification of treatment, or increased exercise.
- To monitor blood glucose levels of non-diabetic patients during treatment with certain medications, e.g. steroids, atypical anti-psychotics.
- To observe and assess patients with certain conditions that may affect blood glucose concentrations, such as liver disease, pancreatitis, and substance misuse (including alcohol), and any patient with an altered level of consciousness.
- As a requirement of treatments that may elevate blood glucose, i.e. parenteral nutrition, the monitoring of capillary blood glucose at the bedside is a quick, simple way of obtaining an indication of the capillary blood glucose.

Professional Approach

- Obtain informed consent and attempt to alleviate any anxiety the patient may have about the procedure.
- Ensure that you have had appropriate training and that competency of glucometer reading has been assessed.

Equipment (Figure 68.2)

- Glucometer.
- Single-use finger-pricking lancet.
- Sharps container.
- Test strips.
- Gauze swabs.

Procedure

1. Assemble equipment.
2. Apply personal protective equipment (PPE) and obtain consent.
3. Check glucometer calibration against the test strips in use and expiry date.
4. Assess the patient's skin, then clean and dry the side of the fingertip, using warm water.
5. Prick the side of the finger using the lancet, allowing a blood droplet to form (Figure 68.3).
6. Apply the droplet to the test strip as per manufacturer's instructions.
7. Dispose of the lancet in the sharps container.
8. Apply pressure to the puncture site with the gauze until bleeding stops.
9. Read the digital display on the glucometer after the required time and explain the result to the patient.
10. Remove the test strip and dispose of it in clinical waste.
11. Document the result immediately on the appropriate chart.
12. Remove PPE, dispose of it in the clinical waste and decontaminate hands.
13. Decontaminate glucometer and leave ready for next use.
14. Report any abnormal result immediately to the nurse-in-charge and medical team to instigate appropriate, prompt treatment.

Significance of Results

- A normal pre-meal blood glucose level should be within 4–7 mmol/L (NICE 2015). Blood glucose should be considered alongside glycated haemoglobin (HbA1c) levels (Figure 68.4). An HbA1c should be taken at 3- to 6-month intervals with a target of 48 mmol/mol (6.5%) for those on diet with single drug therapy and 53 mmol/mol (7.0%) for those on drugs that have a hypoglycaemic affect (NICE 2017). Be aware, when measuring blood glucose, that concentrations may rise to 8–9 mmol/L up to one hour after a meal, but should then return to normal levels.
- *Hypoglycaemia* refers to a blood glucose concentration < 4 mmol/L. This condition requires prompt treatment to elevate blood glucose and prevent further deterioration.
- *Hyperglycaemia* refers to a blood glucose concentration > 7 mmol/L with patients initially being asymptomatic and later developing symptoms (Table 68.1). Hyperglycaemia, if untreated, could lead to *diabetic ketoacidosis* or *hyperosmolar hyperglycaemic state* – these are excessive elevated blood glucose states which, as medical emergencies, require urgent treatment.

NB: When monitoring blood glucose, it must be remembered that certain conditions and treatments may affect the accuracy of the result (Table 68.2).

Red Flags

- Abnormal blood glucose levels must be further investigated and appropriate treatment initiated.
- Bedside glucometers could be inaccurate at low readings – consider hypoglycaemia if the patient displays these symptoms.
- In hypo- or hyperglycaemia, a venous blood sample must be obtained to confirm result.

References

Holt, P. (2014). Blood glucose monitoring in diabetes. *Nursing Standard* 28 (27): 52–58.
NICE (2015). *Type 1 Diabetes in Adults: Diagnosis and Management*. London: NICE.
NICE (2017). *Type 2 diabetes guidance*. London: NICE.
Wallymahmed, M. (2007). Capillary blood glucose monitoring. *Nursing Standard* 21 (38): 35–38.

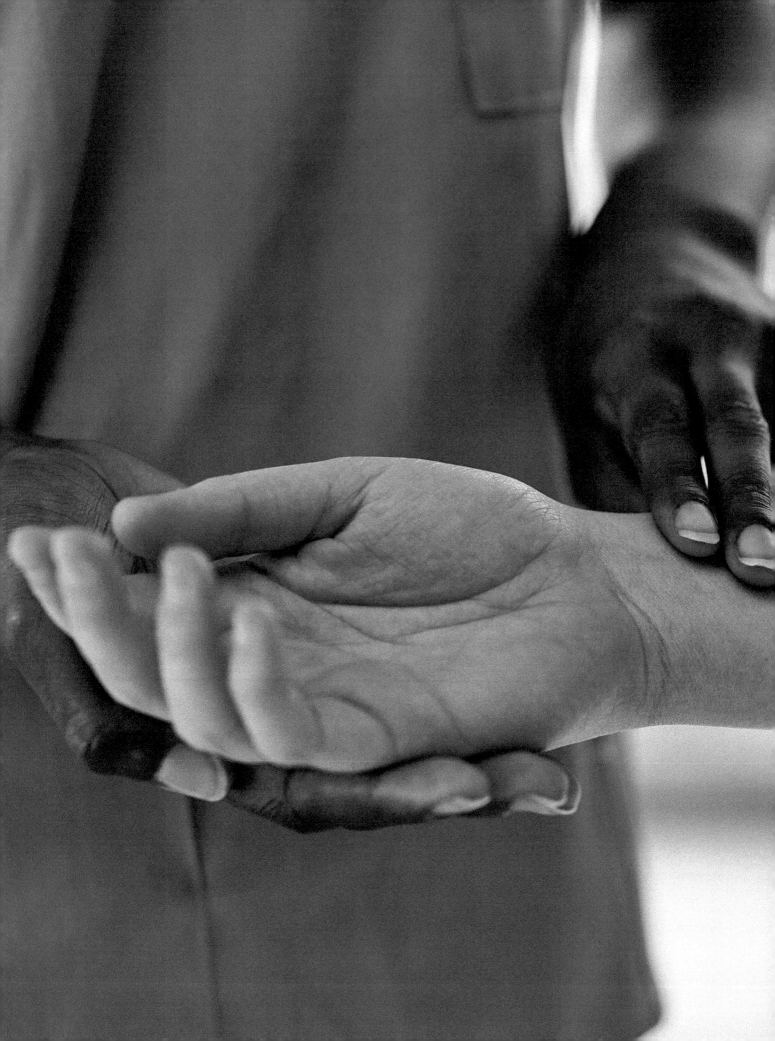

Circulatory Skills

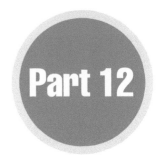

Part 12

Chapters

69 Venepuncture

Figure 69.1   Winged infusion set.

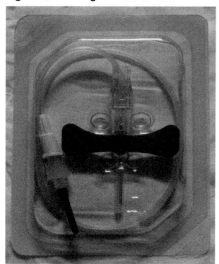

Figure 69.2   Safety needle and holder.

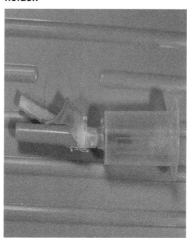

Figure 69.3   Venepuncture equipment.

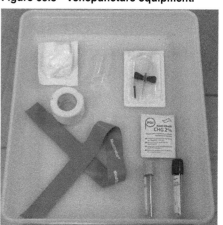

Figure 69.4   Tourniquet application.

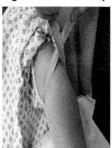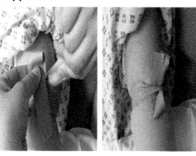

Figure 69.5   Inserting needle into vein.

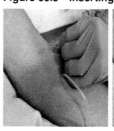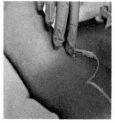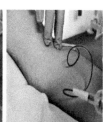

Figure 69.6   Activate sharps safety.

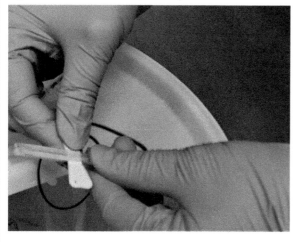

Table 69.1   Order of the draw.

Order	Type/additive	Blood sample – examples
1.	Sterile tubes	Blood culture bottles, other
2.	Sodium citrate	Coagulation, i.e. INR, D-dimer
3.	Serum tubes	LFTs, U&Es, CRP, folate, TFT, lipids
4.	Ethylene diamine tetra-acetic acid (EDTA)	FBC, group and save
5.	Sodium fluoride/potassium oxalate	Glucose, lactate

CRP, C-reactive protein; FBC, full blood count; INR, international normalised ratio; LFT, liver function test; TFT, thyroid function test; U&Es, urea and electrolytes.

Clinical Nursing Skills at a Glance, First Edition. Edited by Sarah Curr and Carol Fordham-Clarke.
© 2022 John Wiley & Sons Ltd. Published 2022 by John Wiley & Sons Ltd.
Companion website: www.wiley.com/go/clinicalnursingskills

Background

- Venepuncture is the process of entering the vein with a needle.
- Understanding the anatomy and physiology of the arm is vital for safe practice of this skill.
- Venepuncture is used for blood sample collection to aid diagnostics, interventions, and treatment evaluation.
- This skill is part of many healthcare workers' daily practice and is recognised by the Nursing & Midwifery Council as a standard proficiency in future nursing practice (NMC 2018).

Influencing Factors

- Critically unwell and/or hypovolaemic patients.
- Those who are agitated, confused, or confrontational.
- Those in status epilepticus or having regular seizures.
- Needle phobia.

Professional Approach

- Ensure that you fully explain the procedure, what samples are being taken, and why to obtain informed consent.
- Maintain privacy and dignity by minimising disturbances and closing the curtain or door.
- Consider potential risks and how you will mitigate these.
- Ensure that you are trained in and competent at using all equipment.
- Remember to follow local policy and consider the person. Two failed attempts are usually the maximum recommended for one healthcare professional.
- Follow the correct order of the draw.

Equipment

- Wipeable tray.
- Single-use tourniquet.
- Single use decontamination swab[1].
- Winged safety infusion set (butterfly) (Figure 69.1).
- *Or* safety needle and holder (Figure 69.2).
- Vacutainer.
- Blood collection tubes.
- Hypoallergenic tape.
- Sterile low linting gauze.

Procedure

- Check rationale for insertion.
- Introduce yourself to the patient, confirm patient ID, allergy status, and obtain informed consent.
- Where appropriate check blood request form.
- Decontaminate hands.
- Clean the tray using same steps as for aseptic non-touch technique wound dressing change (Chapter 63).
- Collect all necessary equipment (Figure 69.3).
- Ensure that all packaging is intact and in date.
- Support the chosen limb at heart level.
- Ensure you are supported, ideally sitting on a chair.
- Decontaminate hands with alcohol hand rub.
- Apply apron.
- Apply tourniquet to chosen site (Figure 69.4).

- Identify an appropriate vein at the antecubital fossa site (inner bend in the elbow; Figure 69.5).[2]
- Remove the tourniquet.
- Clean using the crosshatch technique (Figure 70.6), ensuring that you cleanse for 30 seconds and allow to dry for 30 seconds (Loveday et al. 2014).
- While drying, open equipment and assemble.
- Reapply the tourniquet.
- Decontaminate hands with alcohol hand rub and, once dry, apply sterile gloves (Figure 63.3).
- Remove needle sheath, inspect device for any faults and ensure safety device is working.
- Ensuring that the needle is bevel up, apply manual traction with your non-dominant hand and insert needle at an angle between 15° and 30°.
- Observe flashback, reduce angle of insertion and advance needle until it is securely in the vein (you will usually feel the change in pressure and then advance the needle a further 1 mm to secure).
- Attach blood sample bottles ensuring that you follow the order of the draw (Table 69.1).
- After each draw, mix the samples by inverting them correctly, in accordance with manufacturer's guidance.
- Release the tourniquet.
- Removed winged infusion device and immediately apply pressure with lint-free gauze.
- Activate the sharps safety (Figure 69.6) and immediately dispose of needle in the sharps container.
- Secure lint-free sterile gauze with hypoallergenic tape.
- Label samples correctly.
- Dispose of clinical waste appropriately.
- Decontaminate hands.
- Document your designation, date, time, number of attempts, site selection, and any abnormal occurrences and actions in the patient's notes.

Red Flags

- ⚑ While fist squeezing can encourage venous distension, forceful squeezing can produce inaccurate blood test results, i.e. falsely high potassium.
- ⚑ An arterial puncture will be indicated by bright red blood and should be treated with immediately removal of the needle, application of pressure for five minutes, and following of local policy.
- ⚑ Inadvertent sharps injury requires immediate first aid – gently encouraging the wound to bleed under running water, drying and covering the wound, and then immediately seeking medical advice for a risk assessment; this may be the occupational health or emergency department.

References

Dougherty, L. and Lister, S. (2011). *The Royal Marsden Manual of Clinical Nursing Procedures*. West Sussex: Wiley-Blackwell.

Loveday, H., Wilson, J.A., Pratt, R. et al. (2014). epic3: National Evidence-Based Guidelines for preventing healthcare-associated infections in NHS hospitals in England. *Journal of Hospital Infection* 86: S1–S70.

Nursing & Midwifery Council (2018). *Future Nurse: Standards of Proficiency for Registered Nurses*. London: Nursing & Midwifery Council.

---

1 This could be a swab impregnated with 70% alcohol or with 2% chlorhexidine in 70% alcohol (e.g. Chloraprep) but do ensure that local policy is followed.

2 Ideally choose the median cubital vein due to its proximity to the surface, stationary position and comfort for the patient. If this cannot be palpated the cephalic vein should be used. Avoid the basilic as this could result in injury to the antebrachial cutaneous nerve.

70 Cannulation

Figure 70.1 Cannula sizing (flow rate in mL/min will change slightly depending on device used – accurate information can be found on the outer packaging).

SIZE	LENGTH	COLOUR	FLOW RATE m/min*
24G	19mm	Yellow	22mls/min
22G	25mm	Blue	36mls/min
20G	32mm	Pink	60ml/min
18G	45mm	Green	100ml/min
16G	45mm	Grey	196ml/min
14G	45mm	Orange	343ml/min

Figure 70.2 Closed system.

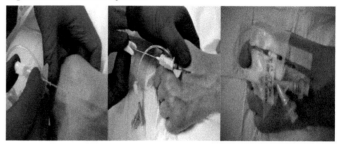

Figure 70.3 Portless open system.

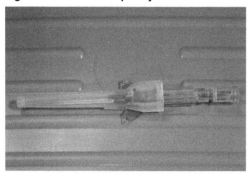

Figure 70.5 Cannulation equipment.

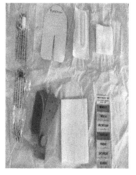
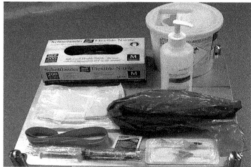

Figure 70.4 Extension set/two-way tap.

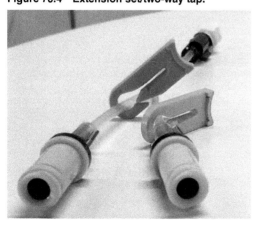

Figure 70.6 Crosshatch technique for cleaning.

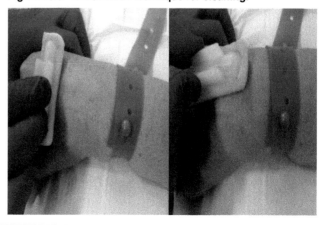

Clinical Nursing Skills at a Glance, First Edition. Edited by Sarah Curr and Carol Fordham-Clarke.
© 2022 John Wiley & Sons Ltd. Published 2022 by John Wiley & Sons Ltd.
Companion website: www.wiley.com/go/clinicalnursingskills

Background

- Cannulation is the process of inserting a flexible tube into a vein, the cannula. The device contains a needle, used to pierce the skin, which is removed and disposed of while the cannula remains in the vein for therapy to be delivered.
- Understanding the anatomy and physiology of the arm and hand is vital for safe practice of this skill. Commonly the veins in the hand will be considered initially for cannula placement.
- Prior to performing cannulation, the rationale must be clear.[1]
- This skill is part of many healthcare workers' daily practice and is recognised by the Nursing & Midwifery Council as a standard proficiency in future nursing practice (Nursing & Midwifery Council 2018).

Influencing Factors

- Critically unwell and/or hypovolaemic patients.
- Those who are agitated, confused, or confrontational.
- Cannulation can be difficult on the following populations:
  - Elderly patients – due to the process of ageing, veins can move as a result of reduced muscle tone.
  - Obese patient – the increase in subcutaneous tissue can make palpation of veins difficult.
  - Intravenous drug users – due to lack of vein integrity.[2]
  - Those in status epilepticus or having regular seizures.
  - Needle phobia, resulting in vasoconstriction.

Professional Approach

- Ensure that you fully explain the procedure and rationale for insertion to obtain informed consent.
- Maintain privacy and dignity by minimising disturbances and closing the curtain or door.
- Consider potential risks and how to mitigate them.
- Ensure that you are trained in and competent at using all equipment.
- Follow local policy and consider the person. Two failed attempts are usually the maximum recommended for one healthcare professional.

Equipment

- Wipeable tray.
- Single-use tourniquet.
- Single-use decontamination swab impregnated with 2% chlorhexidine and 70% alcohol – commonly Chloraprep™, is used.
- Cannulation pack.
- Appropriately sized cannula (Figure 70.1) and either closed system (Figure 70.2) or open system (Figure 70.3) with extension set/two-way tap (Figure 70.4).
- Pre-filled syringe, or drawn up manually, 10 mL 0.9% sodium chloride/normal saline.
- Sterile IV dressing.
- Hypoallergenic tape (in case of failed attempt).
- Sterile low linting gauze (in case of failed attempt).

Procedure

- Introduce yourself to the patient, confirm patient ID, allergy status, and obtain informed consent.
- Decontaminate hands.

- Clean the tray using the same steps as for aseptic non-touch technique (ANTT) wound dressing change (Chapter 63).
- Collect all necessary equipment (Figure 70.5).
- Ensure that all packaging is intact and in date.
- Support the chosen limb on a pillow.
- Ensure you are supported, ideally sitting on a chair.
- Decontaminate hands with alcohol hand rub.
- Apply apron.
- Apply tourniquet to the chosen site.
- Identify an appropriate vein.
- Remove the tourniquet.
- Clean using the crosshatch technique (Figure 70.6), ensuring that you cleanse for 30 seconds and allow to dry for 30 seconds (Loveday et al. 2014).
- Decontaminate hands with alcohol hand rub and prepare equipment using ANTT, ensuring that you flush the extension set, and place a sterile dressing towel under the patient's hand and arm.
- Reapply the tourniquet.
- Decontaminate hands with alcohol hand rub and once dry apply sterile gloves (Figure 63.3).
- Remove needle sheath, inspect device for any faults, and ensure safety device is working.
- Ensuring that the needle is bevel up, apply manual traction with your non-dominant hand and insert needle at an angle between 10° and 40°.
- Observe flashback, reduce angle of insertion, and advance cannula slightly to ensure entry into the vein.
- Continue to maintain traction and slowly advance the cannula while removing the needle.
- Release the tourniquet.
- Apply pressure above the vein, remove the stylet, and dispose into the sharp's container. Attach the pre-filled extension set if using an open system.
- Check puncture site and apply a hypoallergenic, semi-permeable, transparent dressing with date of insertion correctly labelled. Ensure that the insertion site is visible through the dressing and that the dressing meets local Trust policy.
- Flush the cannula to ensure that the device is functioning correctly.
- Dispose of clinical waste appropriately.
- Decontaminate hands.
- Document your designation, date, time, size number of attempts, site selection, and any abnormal occurrences and actions in the patient's notes.

Red Flags

- ☛ Nerve damage results in severe pain. Avoid sites where the nerves run close to the vein, such as at the wrist where the radial nerve is close to the cephalic vein.
- ☛ All complications such as arterial puncture, haematoma, and mechanical phlebitis require removal of the cannula, an explanation to the patient, and management by following local policy.
- ☛ Inadvertent sharps injury requires immediate first aid – gently encouraging the wound to bleed under running water, drying and covering wound, then immediately seeking medical advice for a risk assessment; this may be the occupational health or emergency department.

References

Loveday, H., Wilson, J.A., Pratt, R. et al. (2014). epic3: National Evidence-Based Guidelines for preventing healthcare-associated infections in NHS hospitals in England. *Journal of Hospital Infection* 86: S1–S70.

Nursing & Midwifery Council (2018). *Future Nurse: Standards of Proficiency for Registered Nurses.* London: Nursing & Midwifery Council.

---

1 Cannulation is performed to deliver intravenous fluids, which could include blood, blood products, intravenous medication, and total parenteral nutrition, but could also include contrast dye for diagnostic purposes.

2 When palpating a vein, it should be bouncy, soft, easy to palpate whilst refilling well when depressed. Veins that feel hard on palpation such as tortuous, sclerosed, thrombosed veins should be avoided as should those localised to sites of infection, where extensive scarring is present and at sites of bruising, inflammation or oedema.

71 Intravenous fluid therapy

Figure 71.1   Intravenous fluid.

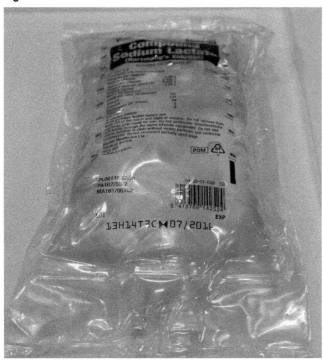

Figure 71.2   Giving sets: (top) free flow; (bottom) infusion pump.

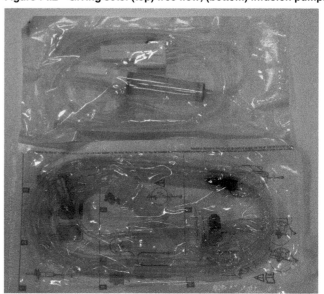

Figure 71.3   Pre-filled syringe.

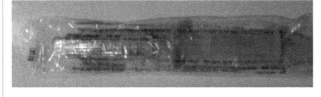

Figure 71.4   Visual Infusion Phlebitis (VIP) score. *Source*: Adapted with permission from Andrew Jackson Consultant Nurse, I.V. Therapy and Care, Rotherham General Hospital NHS Tust, © Andrew Jackson 1999.

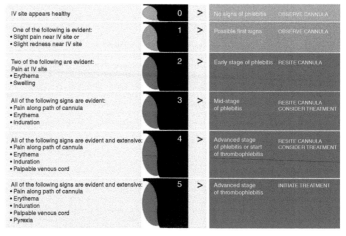

IV site appears healthy	0	No signs of phlebitis	OBSERVE CANNULA
One of the following is evident: • Slight pain near IV site or • Slight redness near IV site	1	Possible first signs	OBSERVE CANNULA
Two of the following are evident: Pain at IV site • Erythema • Swelling	2	Early stage of phlebitis	RESITE CANNULA
All of the following signs are evident: • Pain along path of cannula • Erythema • Induration	3	Mid-stage of phlebitis	RESITE CANNULA CONSIDER TREATMENT
All of the following signs are evident and extensive: • Pain along path of cannula • Erythema • Induration • Palpable venous cord	4	Advanced stage of phlebitis or start of thrombophlebitis	RESITE CANNULA CONSIDER TREATMENT
All of the following signs are evident and extensive: • Pain along path of cannula • Erythema • Induration • Palpable venous cord • Pyrexia	5	Advanced stage of thrombophlebitis	INITIATE TREATMENT

Figure 71.5   Piercing the bag.

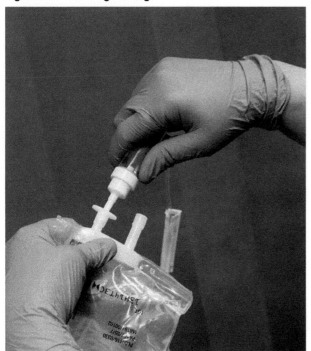

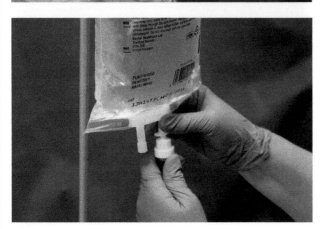

Figure 71.6   Giving set chamber.

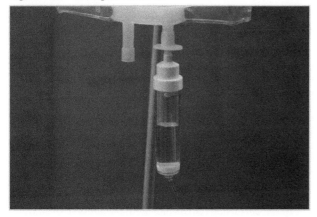

Figure 71.7   Documentation.

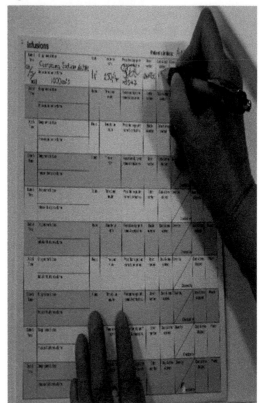

Table 71.1 Intravenous fluid therapy – 5 Rs.

	Rationale
Resuscitation	An ABCDE assessment is used to establish if fluid resuscitation is required. A systolic blood pressure less than 100 mL, respiratory rate of more than 20 beats/min, and a heart rate of more than 90 beats/min (NICE 2017) may be suggestive of hypovolaemia and need for intravenous fluid.
Replacement	Fluid replacement therapy is commonly required in vomiting and diarrhoea, as well as in excessive sweating and polyuria. Fluid replacement therapy will be provided if the patient cannot tolerate oral fluids.
Routine maintenance	This can be required if a patient is nil by mouth or is unable to tolerate oral fluids, i.e. post CVA, in the unconscious patient.
Redistribution	If there are any fluid or electrolyte deficits such as hypo/hypernatraemia, kalaemia or fluids that have moved from one compartment to another such as in sepsis.
Reassessment	Patients receiving intravenous fluid therapy require ongoing monitoring. Once the need for intravenous fluid therapy has resolved, intravenous therapy should be stopped.

Source: Adapted from the National Institute for Health and Care Excellence (2017).

Background

There are multiple reasons why people have vascular access provided while in the care setting. It could be for medications to be given, (i.e. antibiotics, antiemetics, analgesics) or for fluid replacement therapy. The reason for any intravenous medication must be clear to both the prescriber and the administrator.

When considering intravenous fluid therapy, the National Institute for Health and Care Excellence (2017) highlights "5 Rs" to remember (Table 71.1):

R – Resuscitation.
R – Replacement.
R – Routine maintenance.
R – Redistribution.
R – Reassessment.

Influencing Factors

- Toleration of oral fluids.
- Inability to tolerate an intravenous infusion (IVI).
- Size of peripheral vascular access device (PVAD).
- Clinical status.[1]

Professional Approach

- All healthcare professionals providing intravenous fluid therapy should have an underlying knowledge of the physiology of the circulatory system.
- All healthcare professionals providing intravenous fluid therapy must be trained and deemed competent in intravenous therapy as well as trained in the use of all devices they need to operate, i.e. pumps, syringe drivers.
- Local policy for checking the medication/IVI must be followed.
- A full explanation of the rationale for IVI must be provided to the patient for informed consent.
- Check the PVAD prior to commencement and upon completion of the IVI.

Equipment

- Appropriate intravenous fluid (Figure 71.1).
- Appropriate giving set for free flow or infusion pump use (Figure 71.2).
- Medication administration record (MAR) prescription.
- Non-sterile gloves.
- Single-use disposable apron.
- Appropriate decontaminate wipe (for PVAD port).
- 10 mL syringe, pre-filled or prepared (Figure 71.3).

Procedure

- Check rationale for fluid replacement therapy.
- Introduce yourself, confirm patient identification verbally, against the MAR chart, and with the name band, if available.
- Check allergy status.
- Check the prescription in accordance with the nine rights of medication administrations (Elliot and Liu 2010) (Chapter 14).
- Check intravenous fluid to ensure that:
  - packaging is intact.
  - there is no sign of tampering, i.e. puncture.
  - there is no sign of discolouration/cloudiness.
- Note the batch number and document.

- Next remove the fluid bag from its outer packaging and place in the tray or on a drip stand.
- Check the giving set to ensure that it is also intact and in date.
- Remove giving set from outer package and place in the tray.
- Check pre-filled syringe to ensure that it is intact and in date.
- Remove pre-filled syringe from the packaging and place onto the tray.
- Check the PVAD for signs of phlebitis, infiltration, extravasation, or phlebitis (RCN 2016) using the Visual Infusion Phlebitis (VIP) score (Figure 71.4).
- If signs of above, follow the VIP score guidance.
- Decontaminate hands.
- Apply apron and non-sterile gloves.
- Pick up the giving set and roll the roller clamp down to the off position.
- Remove the protective cap from the giving set spike and, with one hand holding the giving set and the other the fluid bag, pierce the bag (Figure 71.5) using a twisting/pushing motion.
- Place the bag onto the drip stand and press the chamber on the giving set to enable the fluid to reach the halfway point (Figure 71.6).
- Slowly release the roller clamp to allow fluid to flow through the giving set. Angle the connector into the tray and once the fluid drips onto the tray, roll the roller clamp down.[2]
- Clean the PVAD port for 30 seconds, leaving to dry for 30 seconds (Loveday et al. 2014).
- Flush the PVAD with the pre-filled syringe using the push-pause technique (RCN 2016).
- Attach the giving set to the port.
- Start infusion either by using the roller clamp and counting the drop rate per minute or by attaching to the infusion pump and digitally setting the infusion rate.
- Check the patient for signs of pain or discomfort.
- Remove gloves and apron.
- Decontaminate hands.
- Document your designation, date, and time onto the prescription chart (Figure 71.7).

Red Flags

- ☛ Signs of breathlessness and/or oedema may be signs of fluid overload. Escalate to the prescriber (or available equivalent) immediately.
- ☛ Intravenous fluid therapy should not be commenced if there are signs of phlebitis, infiltration, extravasation, or pain.

References

Elliot, M. and Liu, Y. (2010). The nine rights of medication administration: an overview. *British Journal of Nursing.* 19 (5): 300–305.

Loveday, H., Wilson, J.A., Pratt, R. et al. (2014). epic3: National Evidence-Based Guidelines for preventing healthcare-associated infections in NHS hospitals in England. *Journal of Hospital Infection* 86: S1–S70.

National Institute for Health and Care Excellence (2017). *CG174: Intravenous Fluid Therapy in Adults.* London: National Institute of Health and Care Excellence.

Royal College of Nursing (2016). *Standards for Infusion Therapy.* London: Royal College of Nursing.

---

1 If the patient becomes acutely unwell, vital signs monitoring and rate of IVI may need to be increased.

2 **NB:** Ensure that there are no air bubbles. If air bubbles are present, run the giving set until all are removed.

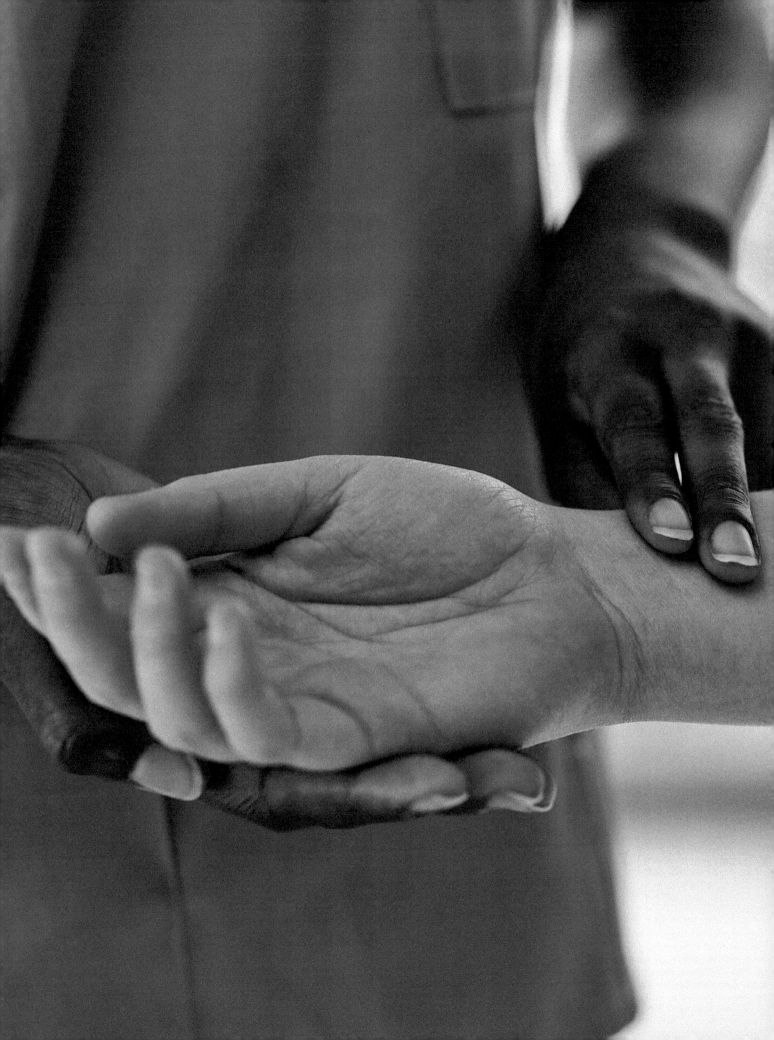

72 Fluid balance monitoring

Figure 72.1 Fluid balance chart.

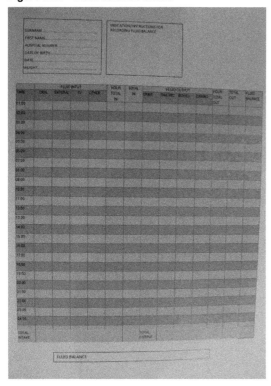

Figure 72.2 Receptacles.

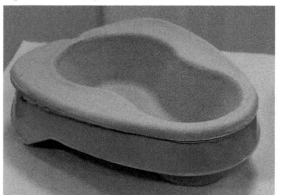

Figure 72.3 Vomit bowl.

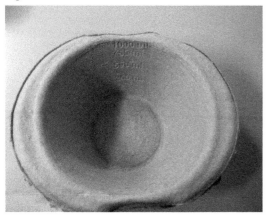

Figure 72.4 Fluid balance documentation.

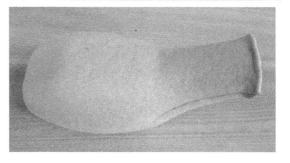

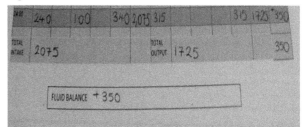

Table 72.1 Average fluid intake and output volume.

Intake	Amount (mL)	Output	Amount (mL)
Water from fluids	1200	Urine	1500
Water from food	1000	Faeces	500–1000
Water from metabolism (oxidation)	300	Insensible from skin and lungs	100

Clinical Nursing Skills at a Glance, First Edition. Edited by Sarah Curr and Carol Fordham-Clarke.
© 2022 John Wiley & Sons Ltd. Published 2022 by John Wiley & Sons Ltd.
Companion website: www.wiley.com/go/clinicalnursingskills

Background

Body fluid is essential to life, with water being a key component in intracellular and extracellular/interstitial fluid (Marieb and Keller 2018). In the human body, an average male is 60% water and the average female is slightly lower, due to fat storage, at 50% (Marieb and Keller 2018). This water is required to:

- Support cell function.
- Regulate temperature.
- Transport nutrients and oxygen to cells.
- Remove waste products.
- Lubricate joints.
- Help form saliva, mucus, aqueous humour.

For this system to work effectively, there must be fluid balance, an equal amount of fluid input and output (McLaffery et al. 2014). While the majority of what is taken in is from oral fluids, generated by thirst, and the majority of what is excreted is urine, governed by the kidneys, there are other factors that contribute (NICE 2017). Solid foods contribute to intake, and loss can be either sensible or insensible (Marieb and Keller 2018). Sensible losses are largely urine and faeces, and potentially vomit in some illnesses, whereas insensible losses come from the lungs during respiration and the skin during temperature regulation (Marieb and Keller 2018). Table 72.1 provides the input/output figures expected in the average adult.

Influencing Factors

Fluid intake and output can be affected by both acute and chronic illness such as:

- Sepsis.
- Diarrhoea.
- Chronic kidney disease.
- Congestive cardiac failure.

Professional Approach

- To be able to effectively monitor fluid and electrolyte balance the healthcare professional must understand how fluid balance is maintained within the body and the processes of:
  - diffusion.
  - osmosis.
  - reabsorption.
  - filtration (McGloin 2014).
- The healthcare professional must also understand that monitoring of fluid and electrolyte balance also involves:
  - clinical examination, such as looking for signs of turgor and oedema.
  - vital signs observations.
  - the taking of laboratory tests, such as urea and electrolytes (RCN 2016).
- Encourage patients and family members to complete the fluid balance chart where appropriate.

Equipment

- Fluid balance chart (Figure 72.1).
- Non-sterile gloves and an apron for disposal of waste products.

Procedure

- Check rationale for fluid replacement therapy and the need for the fluid balance chart.
- Introduce yourself to the patient and explain that you are monitoring fluid input and output as well as the rationale for this to obtain informed consent.
- Ensure that you measure the volume of cups, glasses, and other drinking devices.
- Ask the patient to notify you when passing urine to ensure it is placed in an appropriate receptacle. When the patient can pass urine independently, provide receptacles such as a bed pan, male urinal bottle, or jug (Figure 72.2).
- Check the fluid balance from the previous 24 hours (where able).
- Follow the guidance on how often the fluid balance chart should be completed. This will be:
  - Hourly in the critically unwell adult.
  - Minimum of six-hourly in all other patients who have a sound rationale for fluid balance monitoring (always ensure local policy is followed).
- In cases of vomit, haematemesis or excessive mucus production, provide a vomit bowl (Figure 72.3).
- Where applicable, ask the patient to advise what has been drunk and document the amount.
- Document any intravenous fluid and/or intravenous medication as provided.
- Document any feeds, i.e. nasogastric or total parenteral nutrition.
- Document any intravenous blood products.
- Calculate the total volume in and document.
- Prior to monitoring total output, put on non-sterile gloves and apron.
- Measure any urinary output as per method above. Any receptacle used should be then poured into a jug for accurate measurement.
- If using a catheter, empty into a jug as per Chapter 50.
- If there is any vomit or haematemesis, pour into a jug to measure.[1]
- If measuring faeces, this can be either weighed[1] or measured using the above method.
- Once output has been measured, remove gloves and apron and wash hands using the six steps of hand hygiene (Chapter 13).
- Calculate the total volume out and document.
- Subtract the total volume out from the volume in to get the fluid balance (either hourly or six-hourly) (Figure 72.4).
- If the patient has passed less than 0.5 mL/kg/hour or has other signs of fluid imbalance, escalate care.

NB: Only write figures, terms such as "OTT" or "++" do not provide useful details.

Red Flags

- An increase in respiration rate and/or an increase in temperature will result in an increased insensible loss.
- Wounds, such as burns, can increase fluid loss through evaporation and exudate.
- Oliguria for more than six hours will result in acute kidney injury.

References

Marieb, E.N. and Keller, S.M. (2018). *Essentials of Human Anatomy & Physiology, Global Edition*, 12e. Pearson Education Limited: Harlow.

McGloin, S. (2014). The ins and outs of fluid balance in the acutely ill patient. *British Journal of Nursing* 24 (1): 14–18.

McLaffery, E., Johnstone, C., Hendry, C., and Farley, A. (2014). Fluid and electrolyte balance. *Nursing Standard*. 28 (29): 42–49.

National Institute for Health and Care Excellence (2017). *CG174: Intravenous Fluid Therapy in Adults*. London: National Institute of Health and Care Excellence.

Royal College of Nursing (2016). *Standards for Infusion Therapy*. London: Royal College of Nursing.

---

1 In some instances, there may be weighing scales. In such circumstances, measure an empty bowl and then the full bowl so that the volume can be calculated.

73 **Blood transfusions**

Table 73.1 Blood types.

Recipient blood type	Compatible donor type
A	A, O
B	B, O
AB	A, B, AB, O
O	O

Table 73.2 Signs of allergic reaction.

Wheezing

Shortness of breath

Hypotension

Urticaria on chest and abdomen

Oedema – to face, chest, and larynx

Stridor (late stage – immediate action)

Table 73.3 Signs of adverse haemolytic reaction.

Chest pain

Lumbar pain

Abdomen pain

Loin pain

Oliguria

Hypotension

Table 73.4 Signs of transfusion-associated circulatory overload.

Tachycardia

Tachypnoea

Hypotension

Frothy sputum

Clinical Nursing Skills at a Glance, First Edition. Edited by Sarah Curr and Carol Fordham-Clarke.
© 2022 John Wiley & Sons Ltd. Published 2022 by John Wiley & Sons Ltd.
Companion website: www.wiley.com/go/clinicalnursingskills

Background

Blood transfusions can be administered in the secondary care setting when providing care following major trauma, during major surgery, in blood disorders and with anaemia either due to an underlying condition or as a result of treatment, i.e. aplastic anaemia or leukaemia. As such it is imperative that blood and blood products are administered safely and that the patient is monitored appropriately (NICE 2015). This chapter will outline the required safety checks and the monitoring required during blood transfusions while also providing step-by-step guidance on administration.

To ensure that the right blood is given to the right person, both the prescriber and the administrator need to be aware of which blood can be given to which recipient. There are four blood types, A, B, AB, and O, and while AB is the universal recipient and O– the universal donor, it is important to be aware of other donor/recipient compatibility (Table 73.1) to ensure safe administration (Narayan et al. 2020). It is also important to be aware of the Rhesus factor as this can also affect compatibility (Narayan et al. 2020).

Influencing Factors

As 4248 serious adverse incidents were reported in the UK in 2019 (Narayan et al. 2020) it is imperative that all healthcare professionals who collect blood products, administer blood transfusions, and monitor these transfusions have appropriate training (Robinson et al. 2018). The British Committee for Standards in Haematology recommend that at least one person undertaking the necessary checks has had their competency checked within the last three years (Robinson et al. 2018). This is to ensure that the healthcare professional can recognise signs of an adverse reaction. These reactions can be classified as:

- Allergic reactions (Table 73.2).
- Adverse haemolytic transfusion reaction (AHTR) (Table 73.3).
- Transfusion-associated circulatory overload (TACO) (Table 73.4).
- Febrile – characterised by feeling hot, increased temperature and shivering/rigours.

Professional Approach

Prior to giving a blood transfusion, it is essential that the person is aware of why this is being provided and understands the process. Prior to obtaining informed consent it is essential that the patient is made aware of:

- the risks.
- the benefits.
- the transfusion processes.

Equipment

- Blood product including label and compatibility form.
- Blood administration set.
- 10 mL 0.9% sodium chloride/ pre-filled syringe.
- Clean tray.
- Medication administration record.
- Fluid balance chart.
- Non-sterile gloves and an apron.
- Thermometer.
- Blood pressure equipment.
- Fob watch or watch with second hand.
- National Early Warning Score (NEWS) chart or equivalent.

Procedure – Safety Check

- 60–0 minutes prior – perform temperature, pulse, respiration rate and blood pressure and document on NEWS chart or equivalent.
- 30–0 minutes prior – ensure a trained person collects the blood product.
- At the bedside, check name, date of birth, and unique identification number with patient, on medication chart, on blood transfusion compatibility form, and on compatibility label of blood bag.
- Check blood group and Rhesus factor with patient, on medication chart, on blood transfusion compatibility form, and on compatibility label of blood bag.

- Check blood group and unique donor identification number on blood bag and compatibility label.
- Check the blood bag for signs of leakage, damage, change in colour, or signs of clumping.

Procedure – Administration of Blood Products

- Check the cannula site using the Visual Infusion Phlebitis (VIP) score (Chapter 71).
- Remove blood bag from outer packaging and place in tray or on a drip stand.
- Check the blood administration set to ensure that it is intact and in date, then remove from outer package and place in the tray.
- Prepare 10 mL 0.9% sodium chloride flush or pre-filled syringe.
- Decontaminate hands.
- Apply apron and non-sterile gloves.
- Pick up the blood administration set and roll the roller clamp down to the off position.
- Remove the protective cap from the giving set spike and, with one hand holding the giving set and the other the blood bag, pierce using a twisting/pushing motion.
- Place the bag onto the drip stand and press the chamber on the giving set to enable the blood to reach the halfway point.
- Slowly release the roller clamp to allow the blood to flow through the giving set. Once complete, roll the roller clamp down.
- Clean the peripheral vascular access device (PVAD) port for 30 seconds, leaving to dry for 30 seconds (Loveday et al. 2014).
- Flush the PVAD with the pre-filled syringe or 10 mL prepared 0.9% sodium chloride using the push-pause technique (RCN 2016).
- Attach the blood administration set to the port.
- Start infusion either by using the roller clamp and counting the drop rate per minute or by attaching to the infusion pump and digitally setting the rate.
- Document on all charts as appropriate.
- Continuously monitor the patient for the next 30 minutes.
- Take temperature, pulse, respiration rate, and blood pressure after the first 15 minutes.
- Monitor as required during the transfusion, ensuring that you follow local policy guidance.
- Check temperature, pulse, respiration rate, blood pressure, and urinary output upon completion of blood transfusion and no more than 60 minutes after (Robinson et al. 2018).

NB: Transfusions should not be completed at night unless there is a sound clinical rationale.

Red Flags

- ☛ Stop transfusion immediately if there are any signs of reactions (Tables 73.2–73.4).
- ☛ Never infuse blood through a 22G or smaller PVAD.

References

Elliot, M. and Liu, Y. (2010). The nine rights of medication administration: an overview. *British Journal of Nursing.* 19 (5): 300–305.

Loveday, H., Wilson, J.A., Pratt, R. et al. (2014). Epic 3: National Evidence-Based Guidelines for preventing healthcare-associated infections in NHS hospitals in England. *Journal of Hospital Infection* 86: S1–S70.

Narayan, S., Pole, D., Bellamy, M.C. et al. (2020). *Annual Shot Report.* SHOT: Manchester.

National Institute for Health and Care Excellence (2015). *NG24: Blood Transfusions.* London: National Institute of Health and Care Excellence.

Robinson, S., Harris, A., Atkinson, S. et al. (2018). The administration of blood components: a British Society for Haematology guideline. *Transfusion Medicine.* 2018, 28: 3–21.

Royal College of Nursing (2016). *Standards for Infusion Therapy.* London: Royal College of Nursing.

Index

Page locators in **bold** indicate tables. Page locators in *italics* indicate figures. This index uses letter-by-letter alphabetization.

Clinical Nursing Skills at a Glance, First Edition. Edited by Sarah Curr and Carol Fordham-Clarke.
© 2022 John Wiley & Sons Ltd. Published 2022 by John Wiley & Sons Ltd.
Companion website: www.wiley.com/go/clinicalnursingskills